Also by Frederick Leboyer

birth without violence

loving hands

*These are Borzoi Books,
published in New York
by Alfred A. Knopf.*

inner beauty, inner light

inner beauty,

inner light

alfred a. knopf
new york 1978

text and photographs
by frederick leboyer

This is a Borzoi Book published by Alfred A. Knopf, Inc.

Copyright © 1978 by Frederick Leboyer

All rights reserved under International and Pan-American Copyright Conventions.

Published in the United States by Alfred A. Knopf, Inc., New York,

and simultaneously in Canada by Random House of Canada Limited, Toronto.

Distributed by Random House, Inc., New York.

Also published in France as Cette Lumière d'ou vient l'enfant

by Les Editions du Seuil, Paris. Copyright © 1978 by Les Editions du Seuil.

Library of Congress Cataloging in Publication Data

Leboyer, Frederick.   Inner beauty, inner light.

1. Prenatal care. 2. Yoga, Hatha. 3. Natural childbirth. I. Title.

RG525.L39   618.2'4   76-47945

ISBN O-394-41294-X

ISBN O-394-73459-9 pbk.

Manufactured in the United States of America

First Edition

to Vanita
to B.K.S. Iyengar, her father

to all women
to all mothers
and to the children
who have chosen to be born through them

foreword by b.k.s. iyengar

It is an honor for a student of Yoga like myself to be associated with Dr. Frederick Leboyer and his work Inner Beauty, Inner Light. *It was providence which brought us together a decade ago when he became an admirer and an ardent practicer of Yoga. He soon realized the efficacy of yogic postures and breathing exercises and decided to introduce them to women at the time of pregnancy and delivery. Though we come from different parts of the world, with different ideas on culture and education, we had one thing in common—our concern for the well-being of the expectant mother and the future growth of the child.*

During my visits to the West, Dr. Leboyer saw me teaching mothers, and he discussed with them the experiences they had undergone. He was convinced enough to write the present book, which is the fruit of his vast knowledge of childbirth. When he heard that my own daughter Vanita was expecting her first child in about two weeks, he flew down to Poona and photographed her before and during her Yoga practice, so that he could help all women to keep themselves healthy and to have easy, smooth, and natural deliveries of their children.

Fortunately again, Dr. Leboyer has a thorough understanding of Indian thought and philosophy. He tells women to be courageous and to face suffering, for only then is it possible to eradicate the fear of childbirth and to be free from it once and for all. I have no doubt that Yoga is the golden key to unlock the fear regarding the known and hidden pains of childbirth which are due to past karma and to replace them with unalloyed pleasures.

Dr. Leboyer has rightly said that Yoga is not a dry philosophy but one of action. It is an art and a science as well. By its practical application, Yoga promotes health and refines the body, the senses, the mind, the intellect, the reason, the will, and the very soul. Yoga is an exact science because the anatomical and physi-

ological actions involved are thoroughly examined and systematized by study and practice, observation and experimentation. Yoga affects the mind and the intellect, making one precise, clean, and clear in thought and action. It brings in its wake health, knowledge, wisdom, even temper, and calmness of mind. Yoga molds the practitioner toward proper conduct in life by making each person the lord of his own Self. Hence it is a philosophy.

While practicing an Āsana or a breathing exercise one cannot fail to notice the feeling of well-being that it brings. It is a living experience. One Āsana well performed conveys the entire meaning of Yoga and the real oneness of creation. As pearls are threaded on a single string to show off their beauty to perfection, so by performing an Āsana or Pranāyāma correctly, mind and body are integrated. One experiences the beauty of life and that Inner Light that can never be described.

Dr. Leboyer guides the reader cautiously into and through the technique with a real sense of direction. There is no confusion, and one is enabled to acquire harmony, elegance, grace, ease, and precision. The language is simple and understandable by all. The style will inspire expectant mothers and those aspiring to motherhood and ignite their interest in the practices of Yoga so that they become temples of purity for their coming children.

As you sow, so shall you reap; as you think, so shall you grow. Thus runs the maxim. The key to correct carriage of the body and to the health of the child to come lies in the feet. A healthy body provides the foundation for the mind to function in a well-regulated direction. The child in the womb is the product of the living thought of the mother throughout her pregnancy. The healthy body and the healthy mind of the would-be mother provide the fertile soil for the physical, mental, and spiritual growth of the child. It is my conviction that Yoga helps a mother in delivering a robust and *healthy child. It keeps her body trim and lessens the tension in her nerves and mind by teaching her the art of relaxation. Āsanas and breathing exercises bring expansion and extension, so that room is made in the mother's belly for the child to kick, stretch, and descend. Labor pains become bearable and the delivery is natural. In particular, there is a sense of freedom and joy, a sense of warmth and love.*

If Inner Beauty, Inner Light *helps mothers to follow with devotion the examples and practices given in the book, I shall feel more than ever grateful for having shared in its presentation.*

warning

Yoga Āsanas are not merely exercises.

Yoga is not simply an athletic experience which improves your health. Although no doubt your health will benefit. And even your sleep.

Neither is Yoga a sport, since it is devoid of any spirit of performance, of competition.

The one you confront in Yoga is yourself. All that is rigid and stiff in you, all that says "No."

And neither is Yoga an amusement, something you may play with.

Yoga is a complete approach to life. And Āsanas are only part of it.

Yoga and its postures are a powerful medicine. Therefore, they can heal, cure, and transform. But they can just as easily harm or even destroy.

You certainly would not "simply" buy arsenic or strychnine and "try" them, would you?

Similarly, you cannot attempt to practice postures all by yourself, simply looking at this book.

Which is to say, "A teacher is essential."

Unless this is properly understood, you may run into disaster.

And besides, you would miss the main point of Yoga, which is actually the relationship between teacher and disciple.

A teacher. And not merely a coach.

Body and mind are one. Yoga will affect both.

Therefore, a fine athlete, a good sportsman, or a skilled acrobat will not do.

Since Yoga affects your whole being, your teacher must be aware of both the physical and the mental changes that are bound to take place.

He ought to know the mind as well as the joints, the muscles, and the bones.

Not only skilled in postures, he ought to be a man of high virtue and great moral qualities.

Perfectly honest and true, totally unselfish, and seeking in his practice no personal gratification.

Indeed, he must be what is called a spiritual teacher.

"But where am I to find such a diamond?" you might exclaim.

Indeed, such teachers are rare.

And rare also are perfect, devoted disciples.

Nevertheless, do not despair. Do not give up hope.

The teacher may possibly be longing for you as greatly as you are longing for him.

And it is the mystery of the way that, if your longing is sincere, such a man will appear.

At this point and in order to be perfectly honest I feel there is a confusion that I have to clarify.

It is true that I have been to India many times and that it was my privilege to meet such a unique person.

But the man I call my teacher was not B. K. S. Iyengar, whom I met several years later.

To tell the truth, my teacher never taught me Āsanas.

Or "breathing exercises."

Body and mind, no doubt, are one.

But, in India, they point to the mind.

Once my teacher told me:

"What is the matter?

Never mind.

But, then, what is mind?

It does not matter."

And left me to ponder upon . . . that matter.

Tensions in the body reflect tensions in the mind.

Which are nothing but repressed emotions, products of un-resolved conflicts.

Allow the emotions to surface and the body will be free.

But, then, what about the present book?

Is there any point in doing these postures?

Yes. For one thing, here is a way of self-knowlege.

Here is the strange puzzle of body and mind, mind and body. Are they two or one?

But keep in mind that the relationship between you and the teacher is all important:

blind imitation, neurotic dependence,

or deeper self-knowlege, self-reliance?

There is an old saying:

"If the wrong man uses the right means, the right means will work the wrong way.

If the right man uses the wrong means, the wrong means will work the right way."

Yoga postures can be this instrument.

But much depends on who teaches you and why he teaches.

Practically speaking,

will the practice of postures guarantee you 100 percent security and a perfect delivery?

No. There is no such security in life. Rather it is the contrary.

And, indeed, it has happened that women who have been doing Yoga have had a not too easy delivery and met with un-expected difficulties.

But, yes, the practice is deeply rewarding. Even transforming.

Is it an absolute necessity?

Certainly not.

Should any woman who is expecting a baby read this book and feel:

Oh, but this is terrible, unless I master all these difficult postures, I won't have a happy delivery!

and thus feel disheartened and depressed, I certainly would have missed my point, which is to inspire and encourage.

Hatha Yoga is not a necessity: it is one among many possible ways.

prologue

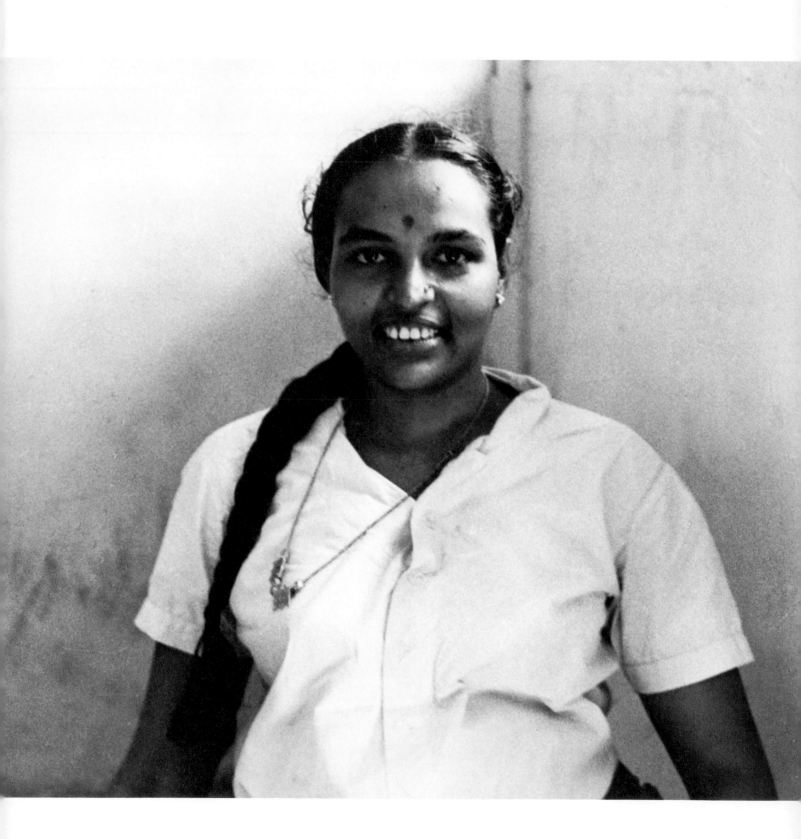

8

—May I introduce Vanita?

—So this is Vanita?

—Yes.

—Who is she, if I may ask?

—A young woman, living in Poona.

—Indian. Yes, I thought so. The eyes, the hair . . .

—Do you see anything special, anything striking about this young woman?

—Well . . . Let me see . . . Quite frankly, no. Healthy and open. Yes, healthy. Even slightly *too* healthy, if I may say so! But charming, of course. Like any person of her age.

—Agreed! Just some ordinary Indian girl. With the natural charm of youth.

—That's it.

—Then, now, what do you think of . . .

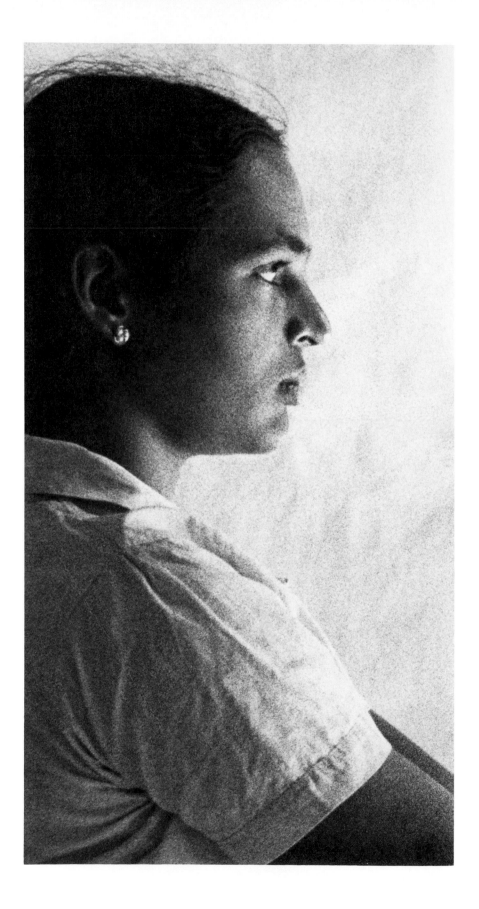

—Oh! How beautiful! Beauty itself. Or rather, Herself!

—Yes . . .

—Not only beauty. Let me see. There is something more. Something mysterious and compelling . . .

—Yes? And do you see any connection with Vanita?

—You mean the young Indian girl you just introduced? Why, of course not. Apart from the fact that they both have eyes and hair and a nose . . . My dear friend, one is just an ordinary girl, the other is a princess.

—A princess . . . !

—Don't you see the poise and dignity? Don't you feel the strength? The tremendous, silent power? And yet the gentleness. Authority and gracefulness. The two opposites merged together. Yes, rarely have I seen such an air of grandeur. And such simplicity. You know, it reminds me of what the Chinese say of the Perfect Man. Although here is, obviously, a lady. And an Indian one at that.

—The Perfect Man? Do you mean, the Saint? Or the Sage? Or the Holy Man as they call him in India?

—Yes. The Wholy Man.

—What do the Chinese say?

—Their definition is as beautiful as it is simple:

> "Sageness within
> Kingliness without."

—Beautiful.

—This is what they say of the Perfect One. The One who is not divorced from the Absolute. The Heavenly One.

—The Heavenly One. Meaning divine.

—And here it is. Here is this "something" which great artists, all through the ages, have been trying to capture and render, be it in stone, in bronze, in wood, in china, in painting. Never have I seen it expressed so masterly, so vividly! Here is no work of mere imagination, no fancy of the mind, no dream. Since, obviously, here is the photograph of somebody.

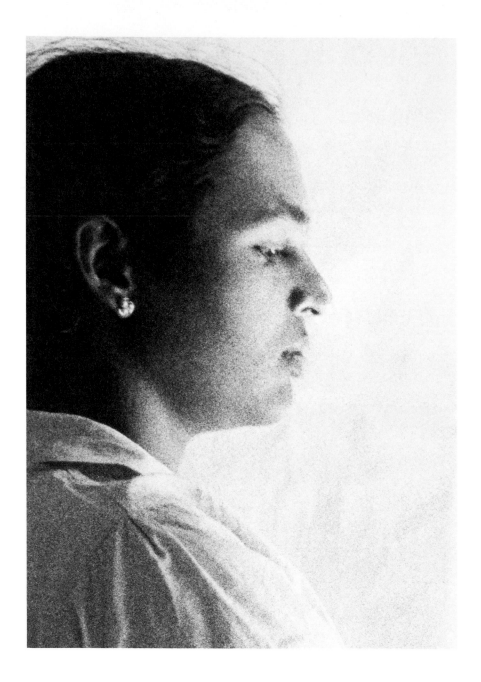

—Sageness within, kingliness without, yes, they are here. But, as you said, nothing to do with Vanita?

—Nothing!

—Well, I am sorry to contradict you: this heavenly one and Vanita are one and the same person.

—Absurd! Absurd!

—So it would seem. And yet . . . it's so.

—But . . . how can it be? What is the trick?

—It is no trick.

—Of course. How could I say "trick"? There is something so serious, so profound. Something that comes from the very depth of being. Here is inner beauty, inner light. Yes, this glow that shines and radiates, this silence . . . This self-assured, this commanding silence that flows so peacefully . . . But what is the secret then?

—Nothing but hard work.

—Hard work!

—Hard work. At least in the beginning.

—I don't understand.

—The secret is simple. Its name is relaxation.

—Relaxation! Is that all there is to it? Nothing more?

—Nothing less.

—I can't believe it. And hard work, did you say? Isn't that a contradiction? How can relaxation result from effort? Besides, relaxing is so natural, so easy.

—Natural? Yes. Easy? No! Relaxing is a very difficult business. Something you have to learn.

—To learn! Can you "learn" innocence?

—No. You're right. Let me say then, something you have to recapture.

—Is that it?

—You have to see what is in your way. What prevents you. You have to see the hindrances, the knots, and then let go.

—I begin to see.

—But, then, it is quite easy to relax on a beach, let us say, with the sun shining, the breeze blowing gently, and a cold drink close at hand. It's more difficult when you're suddenly face to face with a tiger.

—A tiger!

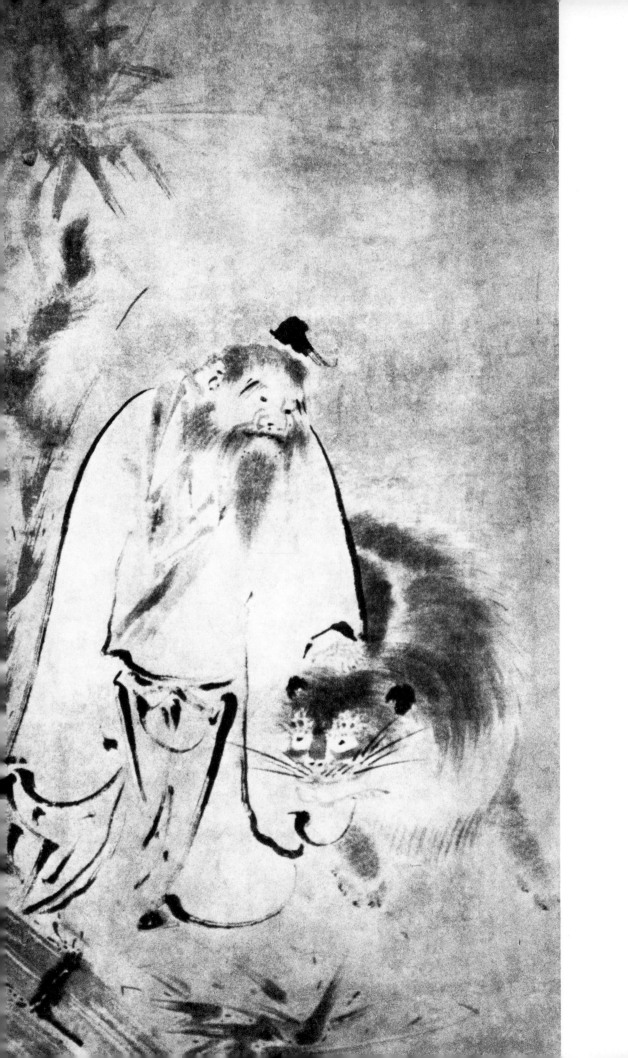

—Facing a tiger in an open, relaxed way is an art.

—An art? A miracle! And what is the name of this art?

—Yoga.

—Yoga! Of course I've heard that Yoga can yield extraordinary powers. Could you, really, with the help of Yoga, master a tiger?

—Certainly. Even master devils.

—Devils, tigers . . . We don't meet them very often these days, do we? And since I gather it takes a great deal of time to master Yoga, it might all be wasted.

—Wasted? I don't think so. For quite some time I used to meet a tiger every day.

—Really! Well, of course, in India . . .

—It was not in India. But let us return to Vanita. The point is that there is something miraculous about her.

—Now you are telling me she is in a trance state?

—She is with child.

—You call this a miracle? Of course it is, in a way. But a very common one.

—The world is full of miracles. The world is nothing but miracles! And yet we keep asking for more.

—But what has the fact of her being with child to do with this supernatural beauty? Pregnant women look simply terrible. Their figure is grotesque, their complexion appalling. And the way they walk . . . ! They can hardly drag themselves along, poor dears, eaten up as they are by the little devil inside.

—In heaven's name, where did you . . . ? It's just the opposite. Through this little baby inside, women get in touch with the very wellsprings of life. They feed on this inexhaustible source through their child. Indeed, pregnancy is the very foundation of Vanita's radiant beauty.

—You're confusing me more and more. And in any case, if Vanita is pregnant, she certainly can't stand on her head and all that sort of thing with her big, heavy stomach.

—That's what you think. But look . . .

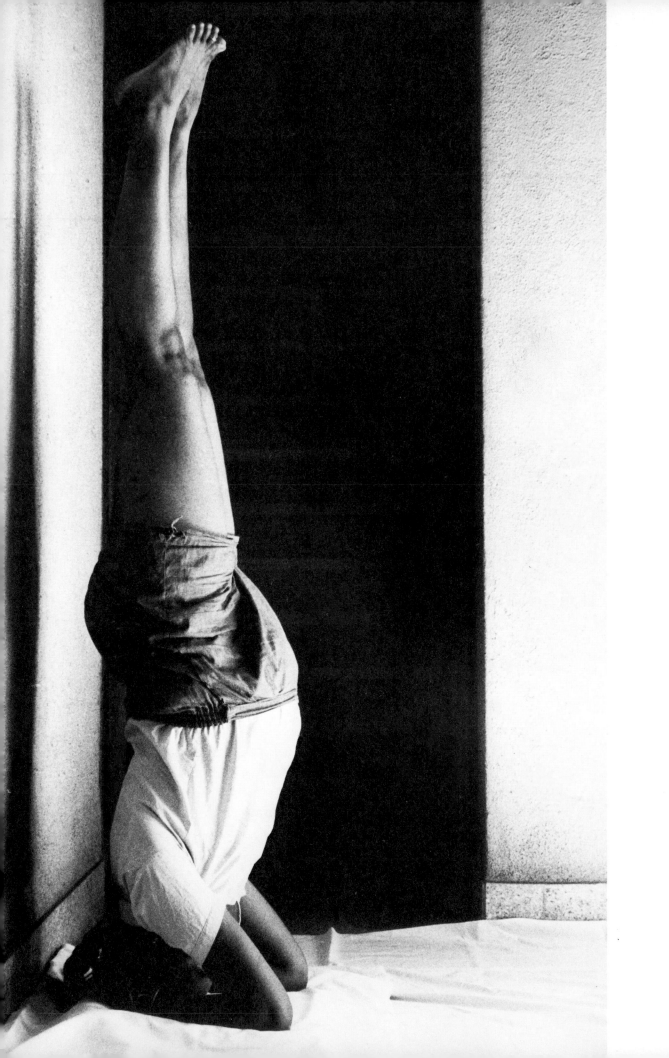

—Oh! I can't believe it . . . And from the shape of her stomach, she must be at least five months pregnant. Possibly six.

—What do you mean, five months? This picture was taken just a few days before her child was born.

—Nine months pregnant, standing on her head!

—But, you know, you needn't stand on your head in order to be a follower of Yoga. Yoga is in very simple things. Things you do every day, such as sitting, getting up, walking, standing.

—Sitting, standing? But . . . I walk, I sit, I stand.

—Oh yes, you do. But, my friend, this collapsed back, this neck which is nearly as supple as a stick or a staff, these tightened lips . . .

—I have to admit . . . But I've had my problems, like any one of us. And here is Vanita and her child . . .

—Pregnancy a problem! But, my friend, you're completely confused! Pregnancy is a privilege. A state of grace.

—A state of grace!

—Of course. It is a woman's greatest, deepest experience. Pregnancy a problem! You misunderstand everything. Now come on. The thing to do is to follow Vanita, to watch her in her daily practice.

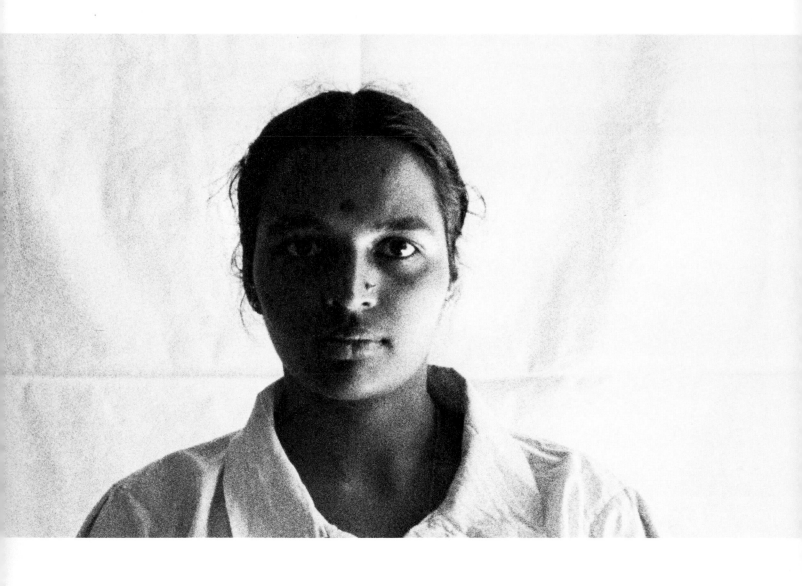

Yes, let us see the fire catch
and then blaze from posture
to posture.

Watch the eyes,
their intensity
and this divine glow
that, little by little, begins
to radiate and shine.

Dawn!
A human being
expressing divinity!

the āsanas

yato hastastato drishtih
yato drishtistato manah
yato manastato bhavah
yato bhavastato rasah

where goes the hand, go the eyes,
where go the eyes, follows the mind,
where is the mind, there is emotion,
where there is emotion, there is rasah,
rasah, the aesthetic flavor

We have chosen to describe in detail the Head Posture, Śīrṣāsana.

Of course, it is not for beginners.

Rather, it is the culmination of the practice of Yoga Āsanas, both physically and mentally, since it demands skill and courage. And intelligence.

And then, it is both an end

and a beginning.

Who would believe that a pregnant woman, with her big, heavy stomach, could perform such apparently acrobatic feats?

"This Vanita must be as strong as a horse!" people will probably say.

Strong?

No.

Actually, Yoga teaches you that strength is not the way.

Yoga is a gentle way.

And a way of intelligence.

Indeed, this is why we have chosen Śīrṣāsana.

For those of you who already practice postures, this Āsana will tell whether your technique, your understanding, is correct or not.

Yes, possibly you could master the Āsana through, let us say, the first months of pregnancy.

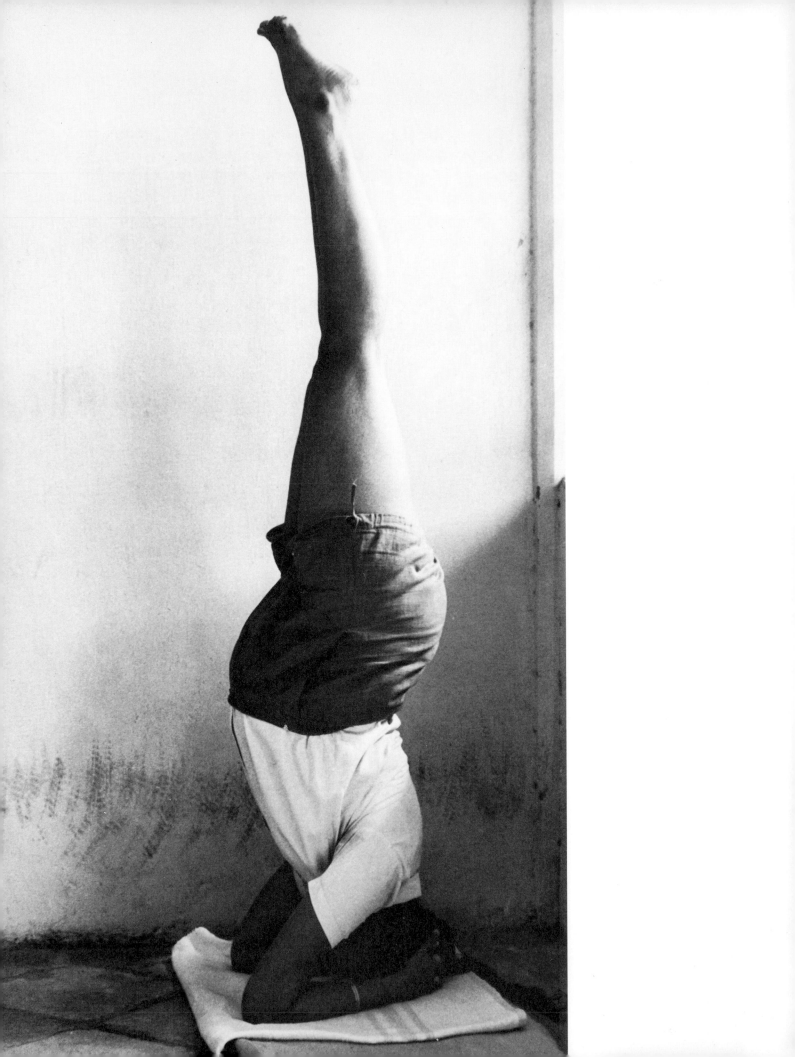

And then, somewhere around the fifth month, you would have to give it up.

"Now I am too heavy. And anyway, it might not be good for the baby."

No, no!

It is excellent for the child. Until the very end. And excellent for you.

But your practice was wrong.

You were using muscular strength.

Which is definitely not the way of Yoga.

Śīrṣāsana is a severe test.

But one who is on the way wants nothing but the truth.

What about beginners, newcomers to Yoga?

Obviously they are never to attempt this posture.

But are they then to bypass this chapter?

No.

Let them mostly look at the pictures.

There are many details they will miss, but which they will see and understand when their practice ripens.

Yet even now the feeling of fullness, of balance, of elegance, the *beauty,* they certainly cannot miss.

Let it inspire them.

śirṣāṣana

going there

Try to find a place where no one will disturb you.

If at all possible, a place where you will do nothing but your daily Āsanas.

Keep it clean.

Burn incense.

And before you enter, wash your hands and your feet.

And your mind.

Put a folded blanket on the ground in front of you.

Thick cotton or wool. But, please, nothing like Dacron or nylon.

Stand up with your feet together.

And then, slowly, kneel down.

Your knees will touch the ground, and there you are sitting on your heels, your hands resting gently on your thighs.

Stop for a moment. Be aware of yourself and of your body.

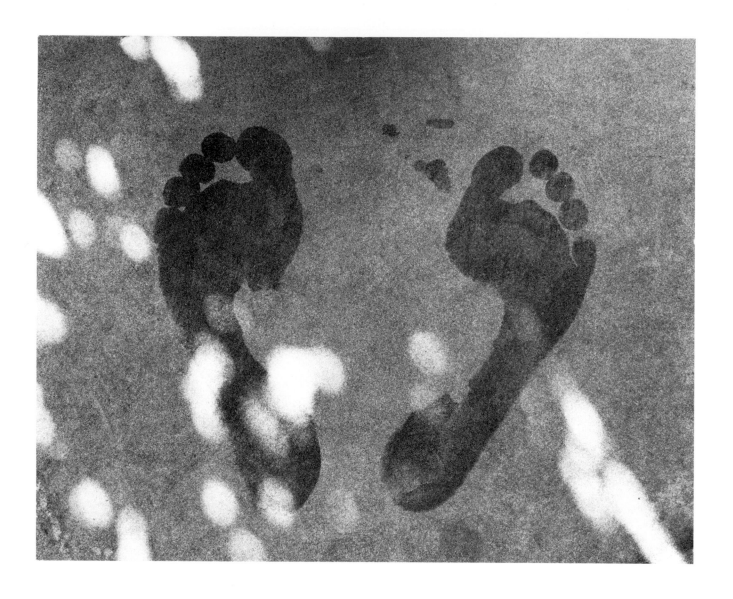

You are about to start on a long journey,
   some kind of pilgrimage.
   And like anyone who is about to travel far away,
   you stop and sit
   before you leave home.

   Yes, be aware of your physical body.
   But be aware of all that is going on in your mind.
   And since as we said, Yoga is neither an amusement nor a
sport, proceed with deep reverence.

And now let us start.
   Join your hands in front of your chest as you would do when
praying.
   In fact, leaving on such an adventurous journey, praying is
possibly the very thing to do.
   Interlocking your fingers, form a kind of little cap with your
hands.
   A cap which you are not to put on your head:
   it is your head you are going to put under the cap.
   Just the reverse of what people usually do.
   But then, Yoga . . .

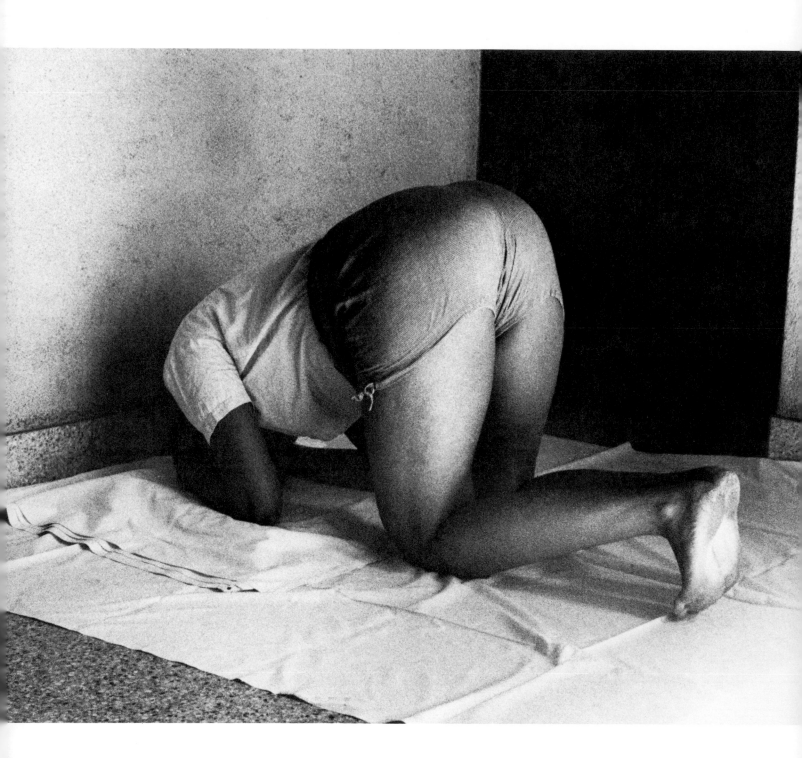

Now bend forward very slowly and let your hands touch the ground.

Forearms and elbows will follow.

And so will your head.

You have been proceeding methodically,

with deep feeling.

Not merely your body, your whole being has been bending, giving way.

It is a prostration, an act of surrender, of complete submission.

Yoga seems to say:

"You want to elevate yourself, to feel great?
First, down you go."

And there you are, like a supplicant, in an attitude of complete humility.

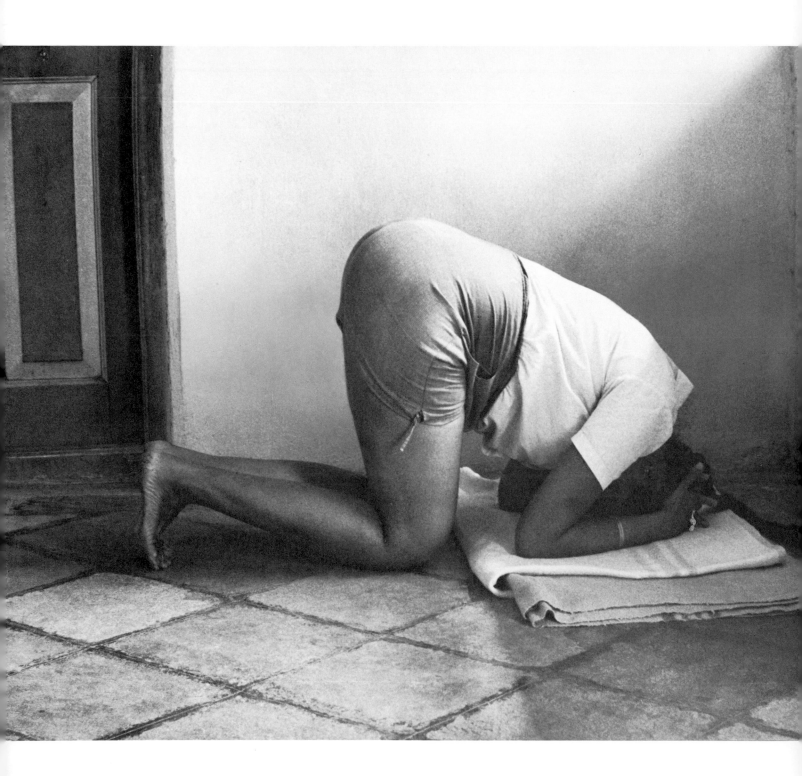

32

But also be very aware of your body, and see very clearly all that is
in touch with the ground:
toes and knees,
for one part.
And then:
outer part of the hands, forearms, elbows, for the other.
Two pillars, as it were, upon which the bridge of your body is
resting like an arch.
Hanging from this bridge, your big stomach.
Inside, the child,
traveling with you
like a little prince,
in his golden palanquin.

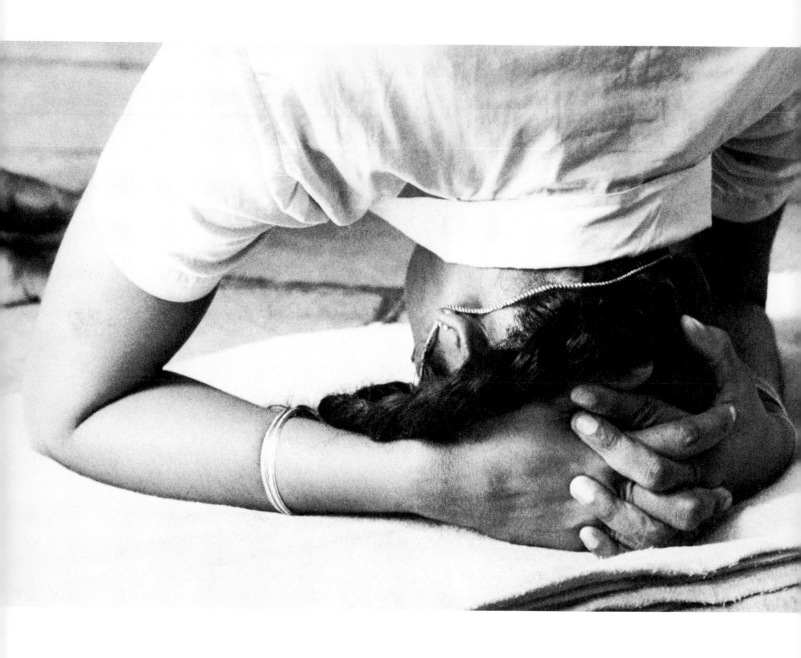

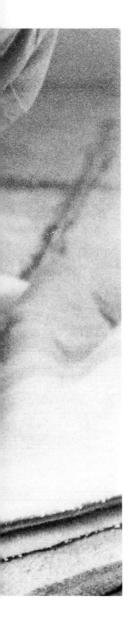

Hands and head adjust perfectly, since they are the key of the structure on which the weight of your body is soon going to rest.

Unless this throne of your coming majesty is perfect, where will you be once you are "there"?

Yoga teaches you precision and awareness.

Therefore, adjust this structure with the greatest care.

It is, you might say, a kind of triangle.

The points are your head and your hands.

Sides are both your forearms.

Check that both elbows are strictly symmetrical.

Not the top of your head but a point slightly forward is in touch with the ground.

In touch.

Which is to say that the weight of your body is *not* to rest on the head only.

That would be very dangerous for your neck.

And you would miss the very point of the Āsana.

The weight of your body is to rest *equally* on *three* points: head *and* elbows.

And since a tremendous force will develop in the forearms, the grip of the fingers is to be made very strong.

Now everything is ready for your ascension.

All you have to do is simply bring your feet up in the air.

Simply . . .

Easier said than done!

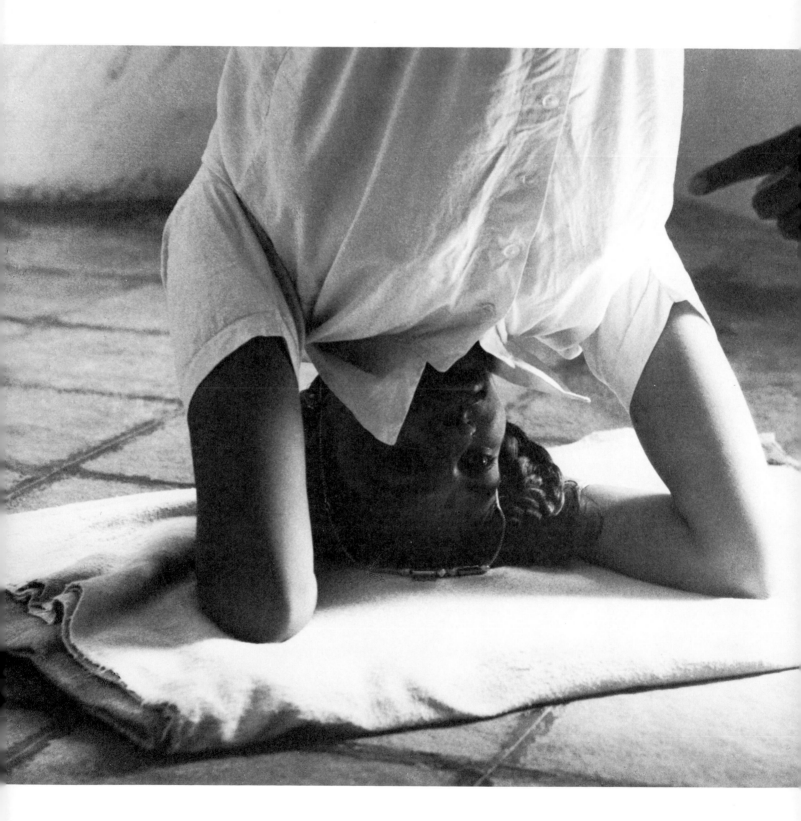

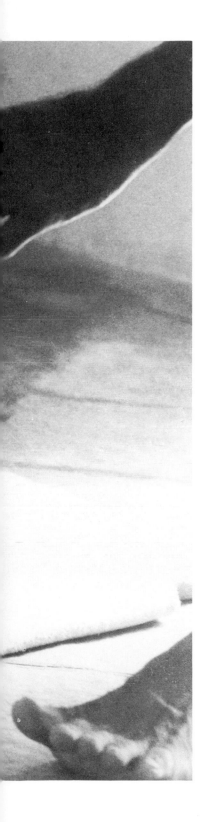

Just as truth is one and untruths are numberless, there are many ways which are wrong.

A natural impulse, for instance, might be to throw your feet up in the air.

This sort of cabriole might work.

One chance out of a hundred that you get there.

And one out of a thousand that you stay.

The next moment, you find yourself flat on the ground with a twisted or, possibly, broken neck.

No.

Jumping is not the way.

Yoga teaches you that you cannot jump.

Besides, you are not alone.

The little traveler inside has also got his or her likes and dislikes. And this little person is definitely not keen on kicks and jerks.

Therefore, please: no jumping!

What, then?

If you are very, very strong you may try your strength.

With a fantastic push on your elbows and a no less fantastic pull on your neck you may get your legs up.

During the first months of pregnancy.

But once your stomach becomes really big and heavy, this won't do.

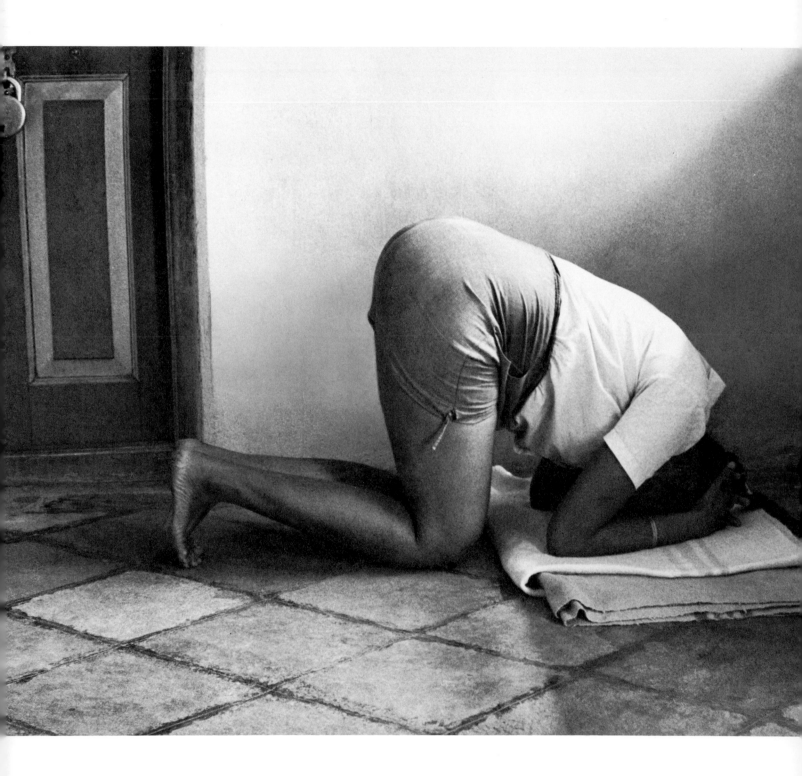

What is the way then?

      Not strength but intelligence.

      And flexibility. And balance.

      There you are with your body folded up, as it were.

      You are going to unfold it, piece by piece,

      proceeding from one equilibrium to the next, then to the next . . .

      Effortlessly.

      But with great sensitivity.

      Sensitivity *is* intelligence.

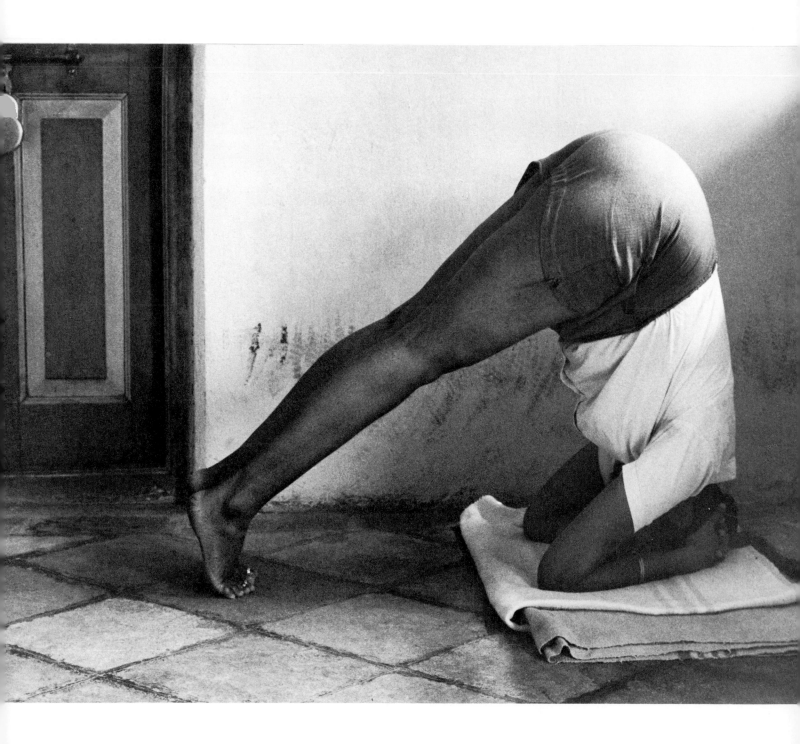

Simply extend your legs by pushing on your feet.

What sprinters do on the count of "One!"

Except that here you extend both legs together.

With this simple motion you have brought the heaviest part of your body, your trunk, halfway to the vertical. You have torn yourself away from the deadly horizontal.

Half the way, half the job.

Then, push on your feet once again in order to extend them to the full.

They were at right angles with your legs. Now they are in line.

You are nearly there, very close to the vertical.

Keep your neck free and press firmly on your elbows.

And there you are!

Your trunk is now perfectly vertical.

He who wants to reach to heaven needs a ladder.

Oh, where am I to find that ladder?

There it is! Your back is the ladder.

But in order to climb, you first have to raise the ladder.

And isn't this exactly what you've been doing?

Now you want to bring your work to perfection. You want this ladder to stand from sheer balance, from sheer verticality.

One more little push of your feet and your elbows,

and your heavy buttocks go just beyond your new center of gravity (which is in your head).

On one side are your buttocks,

on the other your big, heavy stomach.

The whole structure rests in perfect, effortless equilibrium.

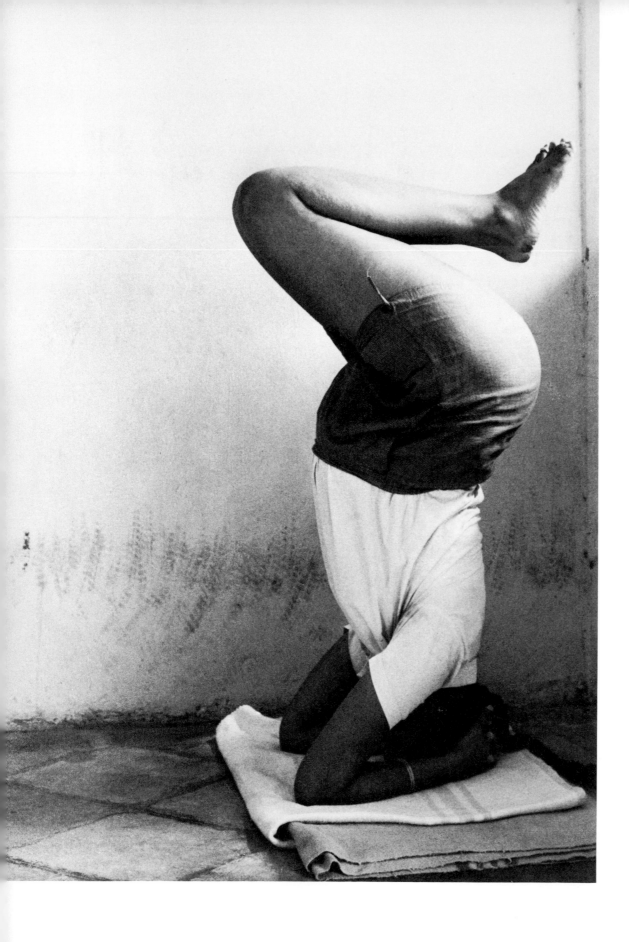

At this point, your legs, which had been hopelessly heavy, have become weightless, empty.

All you have to do is fold them up, draw them up, being very careful not to alter the balance of the body.

Once you have folded up your legs, bringing your heels in touch again with your buttocks: stop.

Check your balance.

See that there is equal pressure on your head *and* both elbows.

This is extremely important, since, as you've been told, the weight of the body should never rest on the head only. That would be very dangerous for your neck.

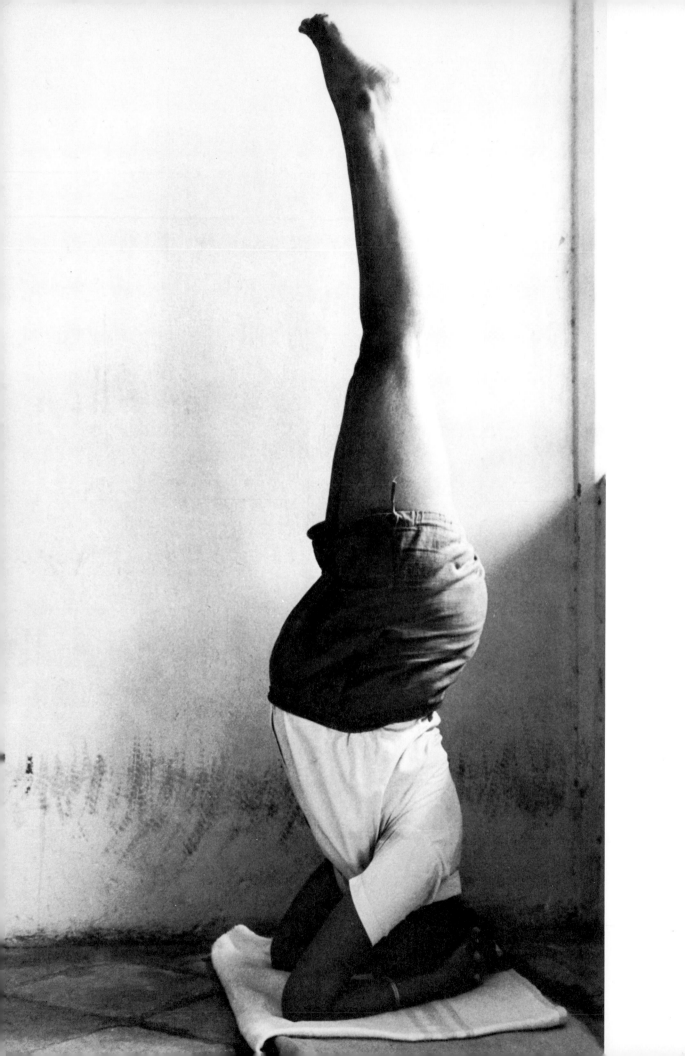

Now, let go!

Up go your feet, effortlessly, along an axis which is perfectly vertical and goes straight through your head.

Yes, no effort!

It is a sort of delightful stretching out that extends through your entire body.

Was this not graceful?
Have you been using strength?
Is this not pure intelligence?

Have you ever watched birds, how they take off,

how heavy, how clumsy they are when still running, wings
wide open and unbalanced?

At some invisible, mysterious point they seem to stop
struggling.

And they are off.

Their feet no longer run. They are very still.

They hang down. And presently disappear.

Gone from one realm to the next, the bird now rests on its
wings

taking support no more from earth but from wind.

When did that happen?

No one can say.

The eye, certainly, cannot catch it, so subtle, so quick is it.

And, possibly, it *is* beyond time.

Yes, from one realm to the next:

heavy, clumsy, struggling,

and, suddenly, weightless, graceful, and free,

carried by the wind.

Is this not what you've been experiencing?

Would you believe the flying carpet to be so close at hand
and that you too could take off
and fly?

being there

For any Āsana there are three stages, three steps:

taking the posture, *going there;*
maintaining the posture, *being there,* enjoying;
leaving the posture, undoing, *coming back.*

Three: Brahma, Vishnu, Shiva.
The ancient, holy Trinity.
Brahma creates.
Vishnu sustains. All that we see exists through His grace.
Shiva destroys.
Without the terrible Lord, how could renewal take place?

"Going there," we have seen; how to climb the difficult, frightening mountain.
Let us see how "being there" feels.
How does it feel, "being there"?
How is the air at the top?
Is it really so glorious?

No doubt that it feels wonderful.
But will it last?
What will happen once the exhilarating feeling of "I've made it!" has vanished?

It all begins to shake. It oscillates.
And then, of course, you try to keep control,
tightening the hips
and the knees and the feet.
Tightening this, tightening that.

Instead of letting go, you add tensions to tensions, bringing into action muscles that had been quiet and free.

The more you tighten, the more you suffer.

And then, of course, the more you suffer, the more you try to counteract with . . . more tightening.

Terrible vicious circle.

Lightness, freedom, where are you?

How long will this martyrdom last?

It all depends on your courage, your forbearance, your will power. And your pride.

Both mental and physical.

Neither of which can prevent the sad conclusion.

In sheer desperation, you hold your breath.

And then, of course . . .

the whole thing tumbles and falls to the ground.

The adventure is over.

A deep feeling of relief. But rather a disgraceful conclusion.

Your construction could not stand the test of Time.

Time, the great destroyer. Our lord and master.

Is this Yoga?

Of course not.

Something must have gone wrong.

Being brave, tenacious, enduring,

yes, this is necessary.

But Yoga is a way of intelligence, not the cultivation of cour-age, forbearance.

And since there can be so much confusion on this point, let us try to see things as clearly as we can.

In performing any Āsana, you will meet pain.

And you have to accept it.

But what is pain?
A punishment?
Certainly not!
How could there be anything to be punished for?
Pain is simply there to tell you:
"Something is wrong."
Which "something wrong" you have to correct.
And you are the first to hear the message.
Pain is nothing but a message, an alarm bell.
What will you do when the alarm bell starts ringing?
Will you sit there?
Will you say: "This bell is terrible. But one has to be courageous, to endure."
Will you not rather go and see why it is ringing?

Which is to say: when pain is there, accept, don't run away.
But don't worship it either!
Pain, itself, has no value.
It is useless.
It is nothing but an alarm bell.
It is trying to tell you . . .

Now, things become clear. I repeat: when pain is there, accept it.

Neither in order to punish yourself
nor to toughen yourself
but in order to see.
To see.
To know is to be free.
Yet how can you know unless you face, taste, be with?
How can you read the message unless you first receive it?

If you merely clench your teeth, shut your eyes, and be brave,
it will never, never help you.

Things will simply be delayed.
Possibly for eternity. If you are very, very brave!

Then, yes; let me taste, *let me see*.
Pain is there?
Yes.
Where is it actually? What is it really?
It is . . . tension.
Tension is pain. Pain is tension. Oh . . .
Then, what to do?
Fight tension with tension?
This is what we ordinarily do.
But fighting back is always wrong.
Fight tension with tension?
No!
Let me accept. Let me open to the pain.
Yes, pain is there simply because something in me is still trying to refuse it.
Let me open to it. Let me accept it totally.
Let there be nothing but this pain.

Then a miracle happens:
opening . . . opening . . .
a deep, immense breath overtakes you like a wave,
it runs all through your body and makes you full as you have never, ever been before.
And then . . . pain is gone.
And gone as well are all tensions that were there!

How could this happen if you had run away?
How could this happen had you tried, as usual, to fight tension with tension?
Is it not a deep, deep lesson?

Have you noticed, also, that we always tend to look at the wrong place?

The moment your construction started shaking, oscillating, you tried to control by tightening your legs and your feet.

Trying to control at the top.

While, most probably, it was the foundation that was wrong: the head, the hands, the elbows.

When a tree is sick, do you apply treatment to the yellowing leaves?

Wouldn't you, instead, see to the roots?

We always look at the leaves.

Is this not a complete misunderstanding?

Mis . . . under . . . standing.

Wrong standing.

And what is wrong is what is . . . under.

Isn't this exactly what happened to your construction?

Indeed, language knows and tells everything!

Foundation.

How is it that the pyramids are still there?

And the Greek temples and the Roman arches?

The answer is simple: no mortar.

Whenever a structure is perpendicular to the ground and stones are perfectly square,

stone rests on stone, effortlessly.

Endlessly.

From sheer balance and the working of gravity.

Why then should mortar be necessary?

You have been using nothing but mortar:

tension here, tension there.

Tension is a hopeless attempt at preserving a structure which is basically wrong.

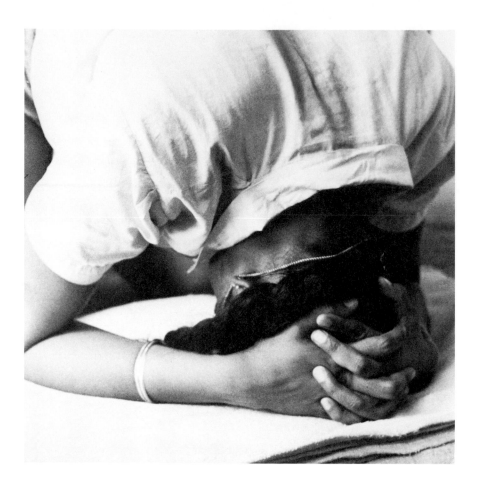

What are you to do, then?
 Check the foundation.
 Put everything in order.

 See that the weight of the body rests *equally* on *three* points:
head *and* elbows.
 There ought to be a tremendous power in
 the forearms,
 the back of both arms.
 The grip of the fingers ought to be very strong.

 Then the chest opens.
 And *deep, spontaneous abdominal* breathing begins.
 Not that you *have* to do deep breathing.
 It is there *spontaneously*.

All you have to do is allow it to play.

Allow it to flow.

Once six deep breaths have taken place, come back.

For the time being, this is enough.

Little by little, week after week, as your practice ripens, allow one more.

Slowly, slowly.

You have plenty of time.

No spirit of competition, please.

Accept your limitations. Do not try to go beyond.

Which is to say, never wait until you are exhausted and let the basic structure collapse and the weight of the body come to press hard on the neck and the head.

This is not the way.

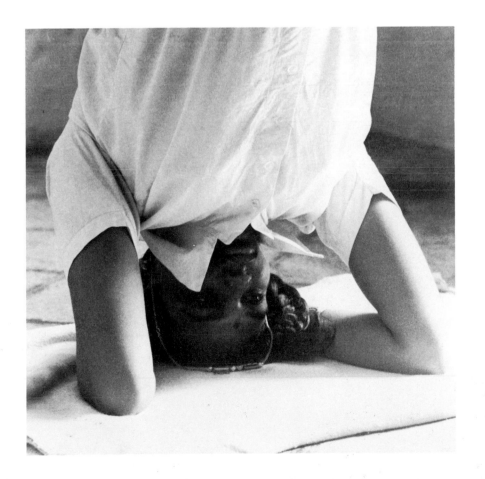

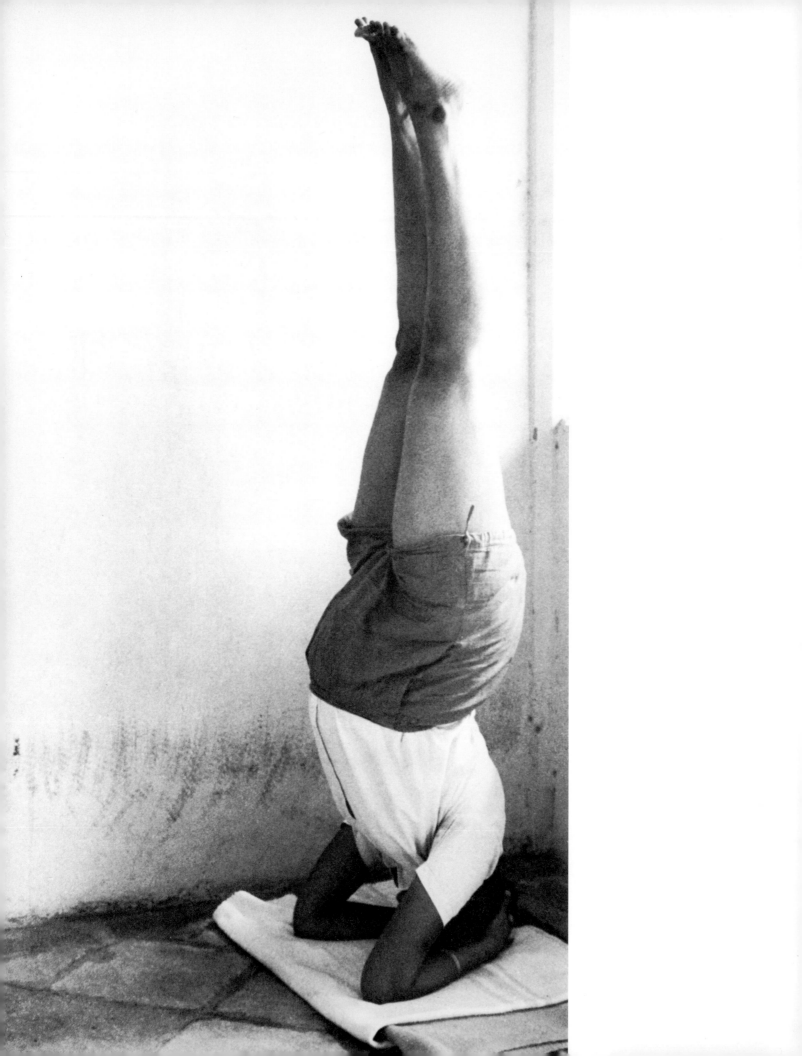

Never forget what Patanjali says:

"Posture ought to be pleasant and easy."

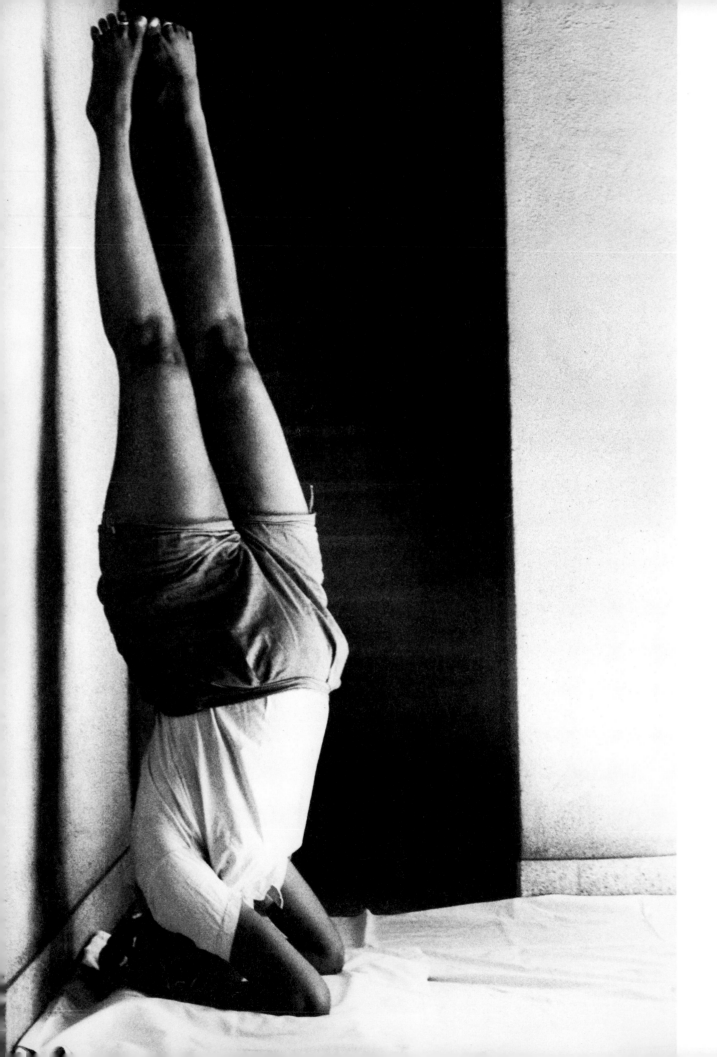

variation

For advanced students only.

Those of you who have no difficulty *at all* in taking the posture
and who can maintain it easily
may try the variation.

It will make you feel more clearly the importance of the *elbows* together with the freedom of the *neck*.

Using the neck as an axis, pushing gently on one elbow while
easing up off the other,
turn the whole body to one side.
And then, of course, to the other.

But please remember:
for advanced students only!

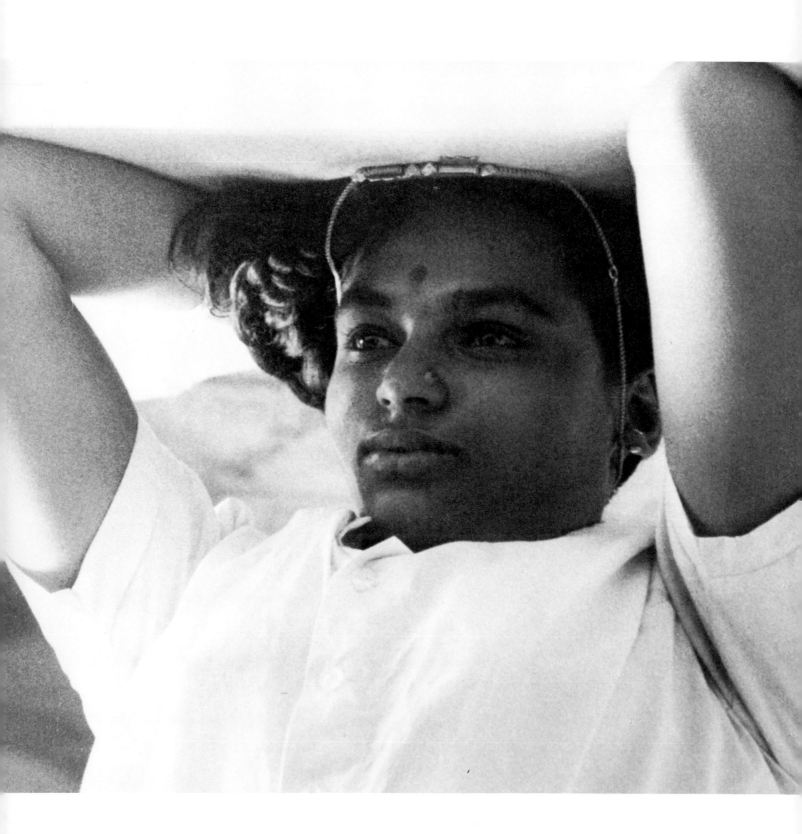

coming back

However high it reaches,
    the arrow you shoot at the sky must ultimately return to the
ground.
    You cannot fly forever.
    Mother earth won't let you go.
    And whatever you have received, you must give back.
    This is the law.
    Therefore now,
    down you go.

Last, but not least,
    coming back, parting with elegance, is not easy.
    Any pilot will tell you that compared with landing, flying is
child's play.
    Yes, landing is the difficulty.
    It is there that your skill, your mastery, will show.

Retracing your steps,
    you visit again the places you have known
    and enjoyed, the places you reached, at times,
    with great difficulty.
    Again you meet your joys. And your sorrows. And your sur-
prises.
    But all along now
    your face remains quiet,
    peaceful, happy.

Falling down is, of course, out of the question.

You are to come down very, very slowly, in complete command and control of the whole journey,

fully aware of all that is going on,

of where you are and where you want to go,

moving from place to place at your will

and undoing the construction methodically, piece by piece.

While nothing else moves in your body,

first bring the feet down.

The knees follow, folding,

and your feet, once again, come to rest on top of your buttocks.

The trunk is still perfectly vertical.

Stop.

With folded limbs and head pressing hard on the ground

(and at this very point you may allow the weight of the body to rest entirely on the head),

how does it feel?

And do you know what you really look like?

You look exactly . . . like the child within, about to be born, working its way through the pangs of labor!

What you are experiencing right now is what you went through long, long ago when

you

were born.

Strange, isn't it?

But now you know.

And knowing makes you free.

And while you are re-experiencing the terrible pressure, the squeezing,

the child within you, on the contrary, suddenly feels free.

For this little baby, no more pressure on the head. Which at the moment is just opposite yours.

Who can doubt that this little one enjoys the Āsana immensely?

One of you head down and the other with its head at the top, aren't you just like the figures on playing cards?
Jack of hearts? Or the queen?

The two of you on the same path,
walking in opposite directions.
One is going, one is coming.
And yet both of you
going to reach and meet at the very same place!

Once you have seen through and through all that is going on,
once you have felt each and every bone along your back,
along your neck,
and each and every spot along your spine,
and felt the tremendous pressure on the head and seen what
it meant,
once you have seen how the flexibility of the neck, and freedom and openness of breathing
can make it all so easy and yet so rich,
so fantastic,
come down.
Live, once again, with gravity.
Allow mother earth, once again, to carry you.

Now you may land:
there is a kind of letting go in the lower part of your back,
and in your neck,

and a bending forward in the lower part of your body.

Your elbows keep control and see to it that everything goes slowly and gently.

Your empty legs unfold.

Your feet touch the ground.

Then the legs fold up again while your knees touch the ground.

And, the next moment, your body comes down altogether, your buttocks rest again on your heels.

Keep your head down!

Indeed, this is extremely important.

When you were born you were handled so roughly!

At least this time be born gently, properly.

Allow the transition to be very slow, so that you can enjoy each and every step of the whole process.

Feel the long, deep, easy, happy breath which runs through you, opening your back from bottom to the neck.

Did you ever experience before such deep, fulfilling breathing?

Yes, let go. Relax. Enjoy.

It's all over.

You are born.

And then, with your head still in touch with the ground, stretch out both your arms.

Allow both your hands to go forward as far as they can reach.

Yes, stretch out from the tip of your fingers to the small of your back.

With the ease and sheer delight that only cats can enjoy.

And now come back once more, part with the horizontal, sit again.

But again, you are to do this very, very slowly.

Try to feel that it is not *your doing,* but rather that it *simply happens.*

The movement starts, as it were, in the small of the back.

There is a kind of pull that comes from your buttocks and from your heels.

Your back is like some kind of whip.

Or like a young bamboo once curved by a powerful wind and now released.

For, yes, the storm is over now.

As your back unfolds, your hands come to rest gently on your thighs.

They come? No. Once again, they have been drawn back passively, caressing the ground all the way with great sensitivity.

And last goes your head, which has remained hanging forward till the very end.

Yes, the head goes up only when the back is straight again.

There you are, sitting quietly on your heels again.

Take rest.

Don't move.

And . . .

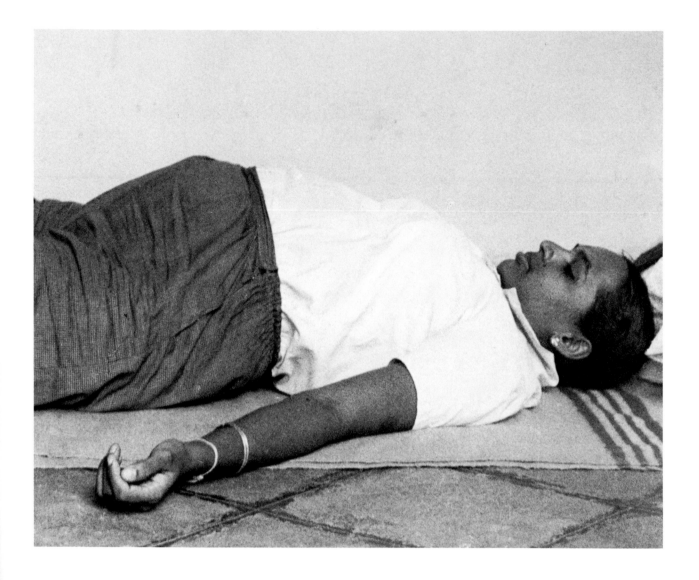

Before you proceed with any of the other Āsanas, you are to lie down and rest.

This is extremely important.

You are not to lie flat on your back,

but you should use a pillow, as is explained in greater detail with Supta Vīrāsana (p. 159) and Śavāsana (p. 167).

If you compare the two pictures, you can see that when you lie flat on your back there can be no freedom in your neck, in your shoulders, or in your chest.

See how the chest is open in the lower picture.

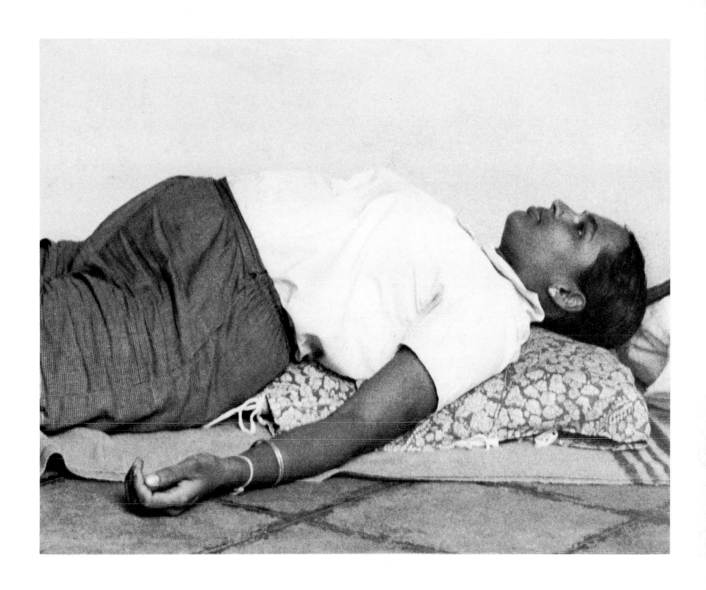

How does it feel
to be born?
For, indeed, this full breath,
this tidal wave which, starting in the belly,
sweeps over,
making you feel drunk and dizzy,
is it not the way it feels
to the baby
making its entrance
into this oscillating, pulsating world
we call life?

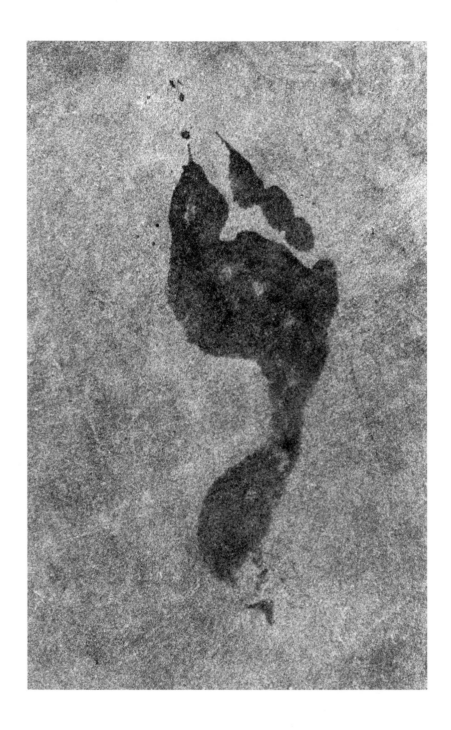

It has been a long way.
And yet you did not move an inch.

There you are again
on your heels,
sitting peacefully.

A long way
from your heels
to your toes.

A long, long way.

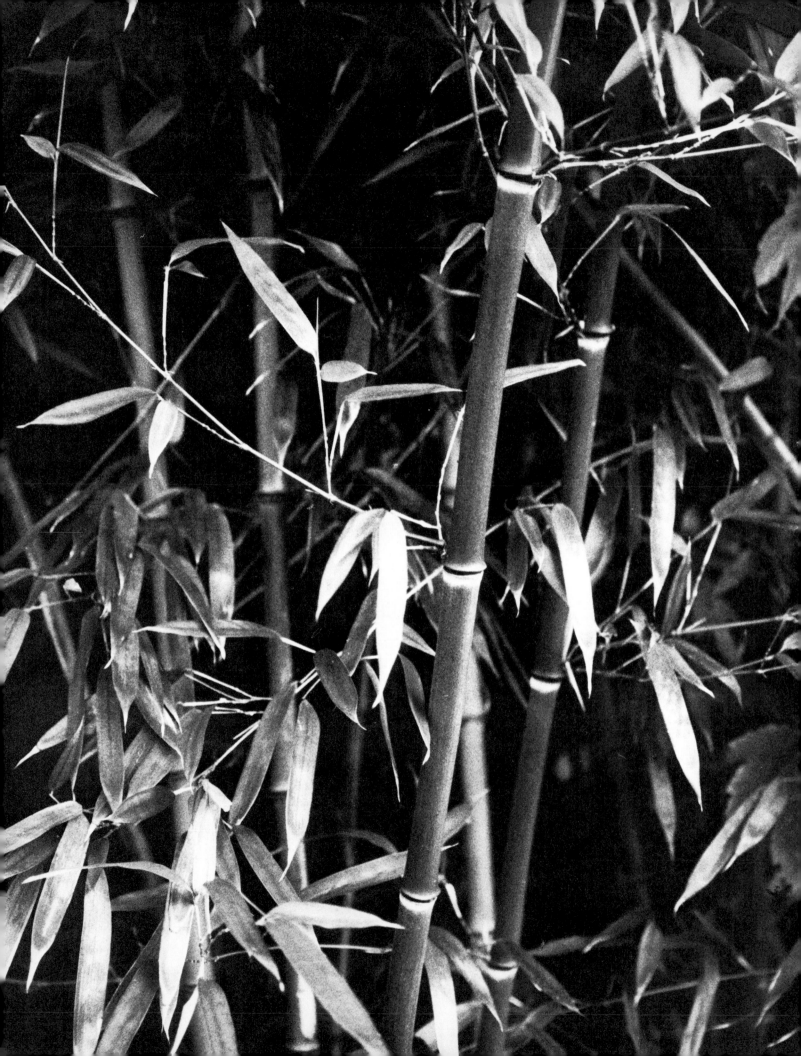

What has happened?
Nothing, in a way.

But who had expected
the roots of this graceful bamboo
to be so strong
to go so deep?

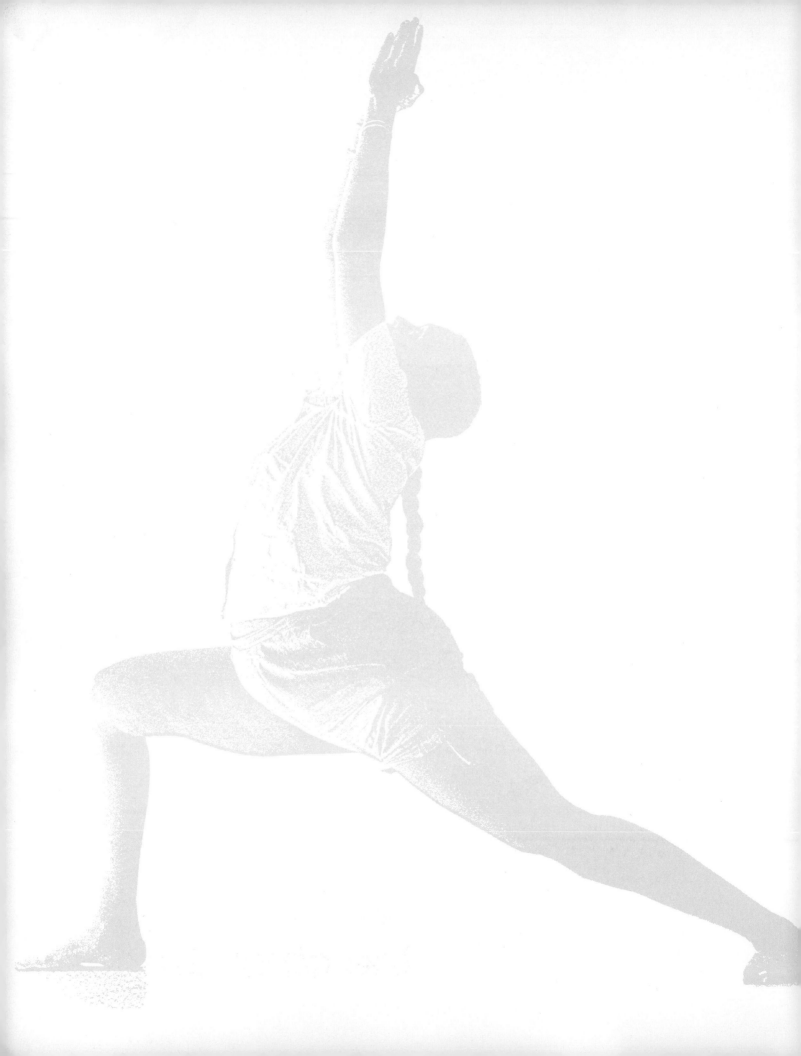

the other āsanas

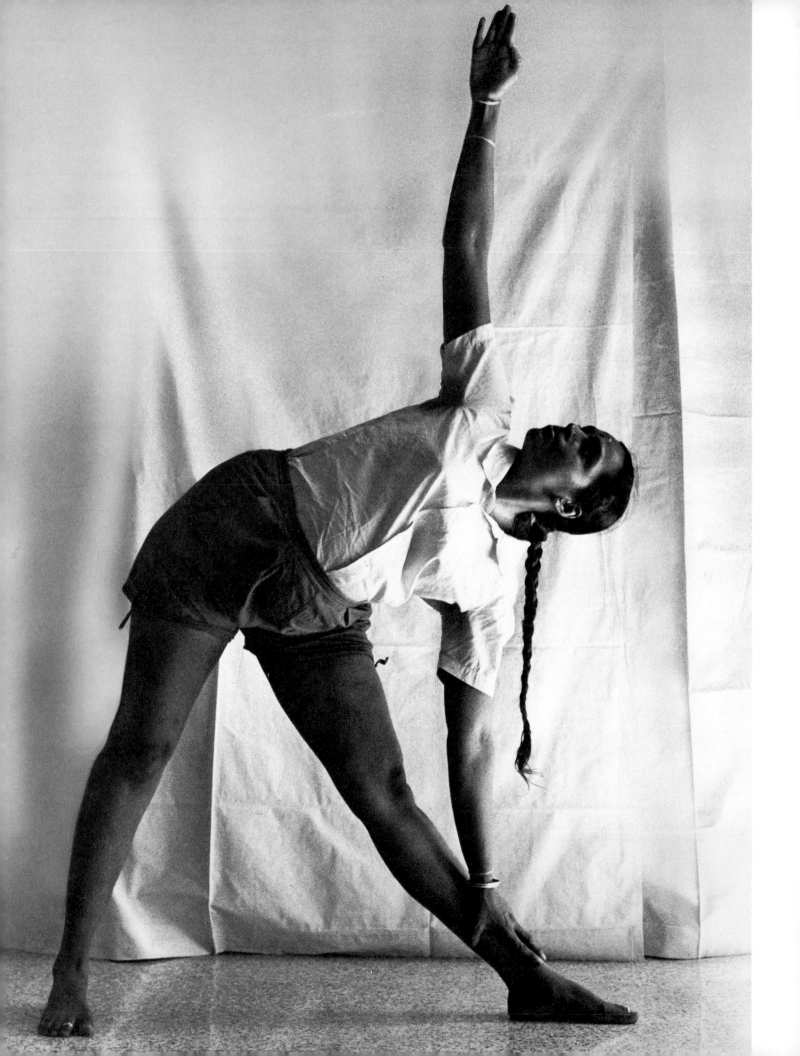

Now you may proceed to the other Āsanas.

Whether you are to perform all of them is a point we shall discuss later.

uttihita trikoṇāṣana

Here is the first of the *standing postures* which you may perform until the very end of pregnancy.

You may notice many triangles.

Could the Creator, Brahma, be a *great architect,* taking delight in geometry?

And is not Yoga *geometry in action?*

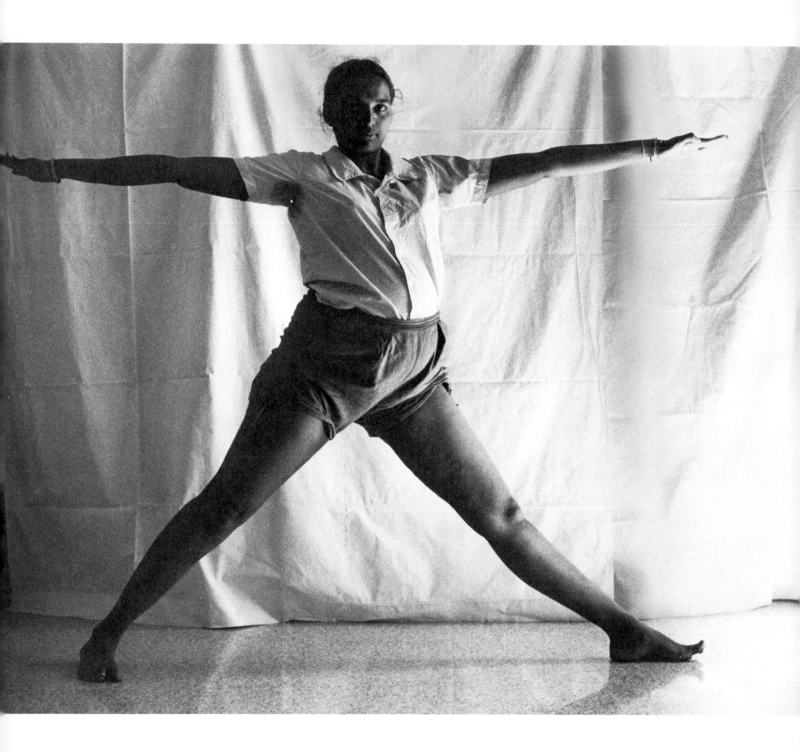

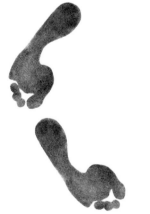

1

2

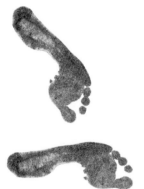

Once again, notice the importance of the feet.
Right basis, right foundation!

Start feet apart, your legs forming a perfect triangle.
Your feet are on one line, which we might call A – B.
And you will move your feet from position 1 to position 2.
Simply by *pivoting* on your *heels*.

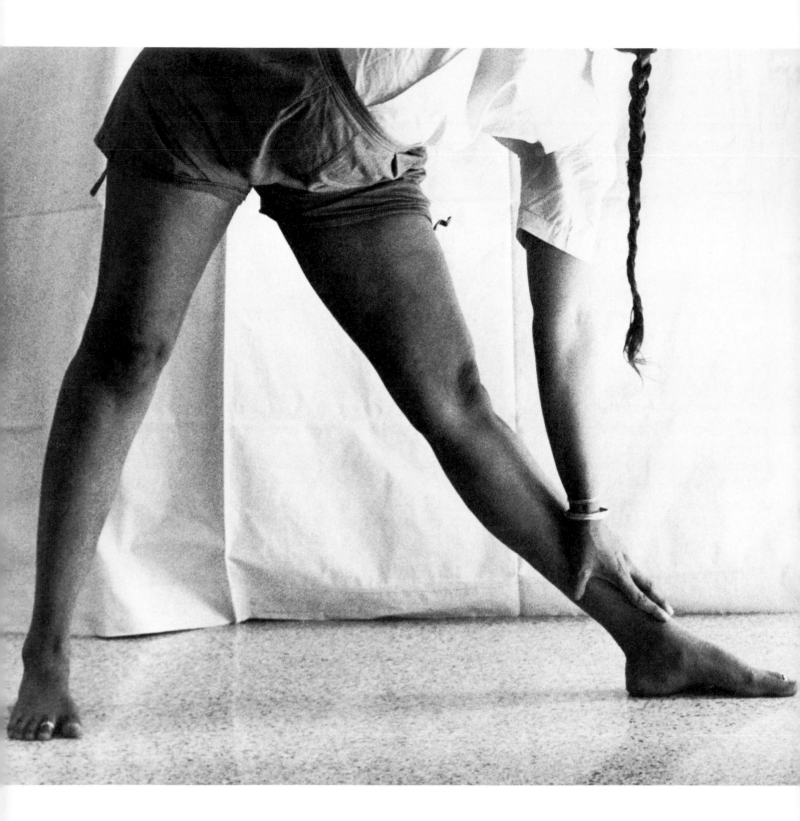

Then, keeping hips and pelvis motionless, the trunk starts its motion sideways.

How are you to reach there?

All at once?

No.

You are to progress slowly, *in tune with your breathing*.

For, as always, breathing is the secret.

And thinking!

Thinking of your lower hand, try to reach a little lower as you *exhale*.

When you start to *inhale*, shift your mind to the upper hand and, stretching, try to reach a little higher.

When you next *exhale*, shift the mind again to the lower hand . . .

Stretching! Stretching! Trying to create as much distance and space between your two hands as possible.

Always remember:

inhaling should never be *your* doing.

It must be kept passive.

It is the spontaneous response to *exhaling*.

With *exhaling* you may work.

In this Āsana, when you try to reach farther and farther with your lower hand,

you progress with *exhaling*.

When you are totally empty, inhaling takes place,

suddenly, spontaneously, and fills you.

"Empty, empty!" says Yoga. "Give, give!"

For, indeed, giving is getting.

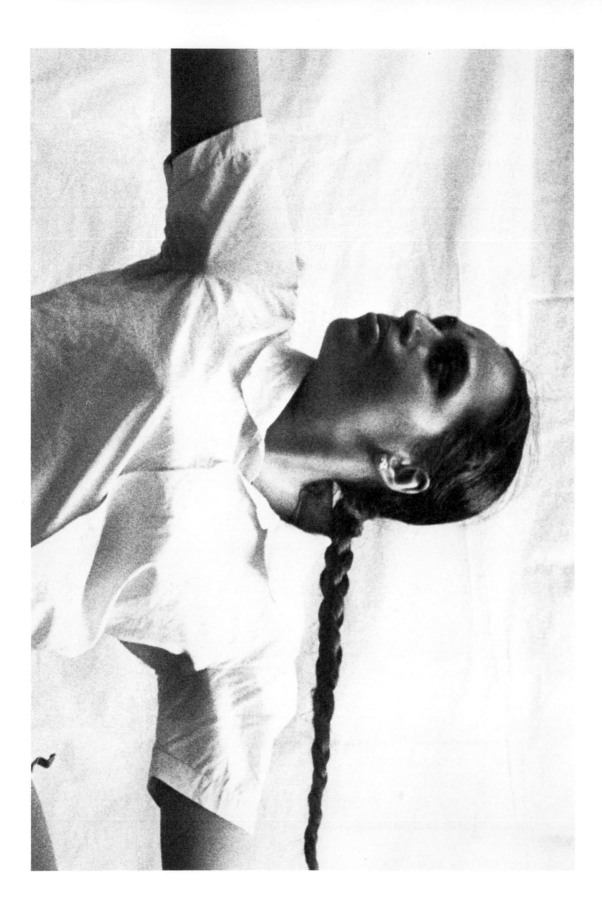

Driven by the *eyes,* which you are to keep constantly focused on the *upper* hand, the head turns forcibly.

> "Where goes the hand
> there go the eyes,
> where go the eyes
> there goes the mind . . ."

So you are to guide your mind constantly and learn to bring it where you want: here, and there, and there . . .

But the eyes are never to move away from the upper hand.

Yet be constantly watchful of the shift of the mind from *right* to *left,* from *left* to *right,*

from *lower* hand to *upper* hand, then back to lower hand . . .

moving always together with . . . breathing.

And be careful that your mind does not fly away . . . to the sky!

Yes, keep it on your hand!

A few important points:

legs are to be absolutely straight. No bending at the knees!

Arms are to be strictly on *one line* and perpendicular to the ground.

But the main point is that the pelvis should not move.

Should it rotate, the Āsana becomes much, much easier. But at the same time the entire benefit vanishes.

In order to prevent this rotation, practice along a wall and very close to it.

The moment the pelvis starts rotating, one buttock moves backward,

which it should not do.

The wall will stop it and prevent the mistake.

Pelvis and buttocks are to remain strictly parallel to the line which is uniting your feet, A – B.

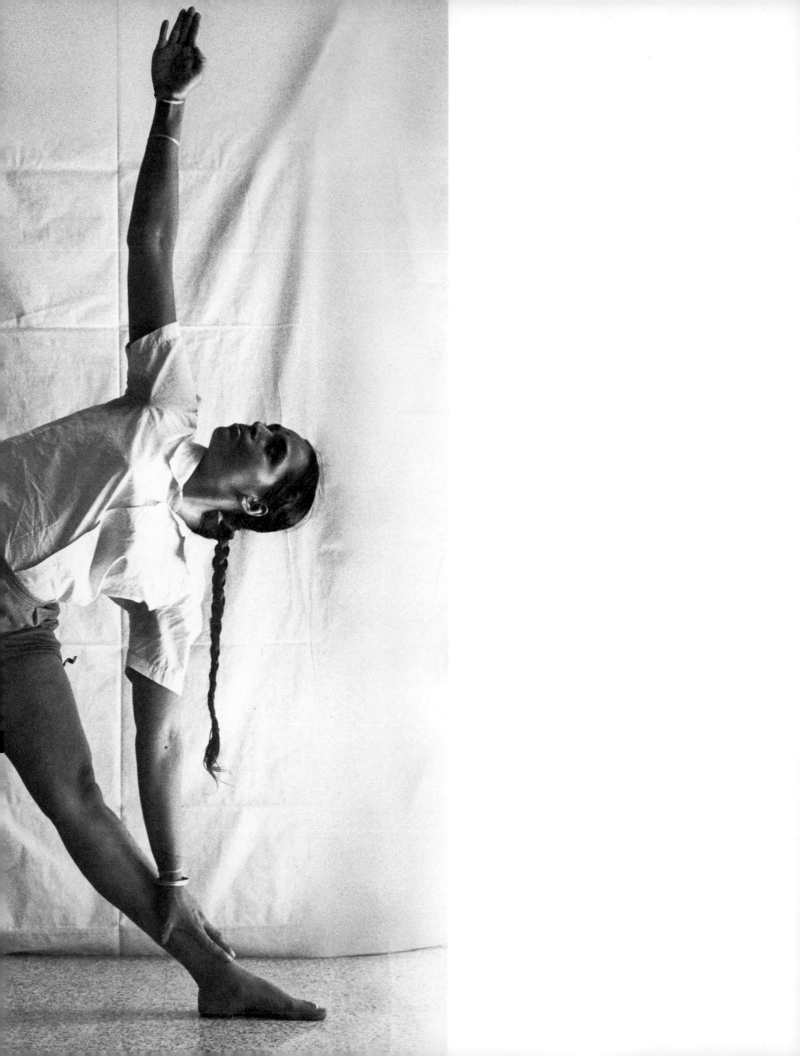

"Then came Rama.
    And he took Govinda, the mighty bow, which
none of the other princes could even lift,
        and, effortlessly, strung it!"

                        Ramayana

"But Odysseus, the wise one, took the bow which
    none of the other princes could string, using
all their might,
        and, with the same ease with which a
musician strings his lyre,
        Odysseus, effortlessly, strung the mighty bow.
        Rather he merely tried the string and let go.
        A beautiful sound was heard,
        as clear and gay as the song of the morning lark.
        And at the very same moment,
        like an echo,
        thunder!
        Which Zeus, son of Cronus,
        as an answer, also let go!

                        —Odyssey XXI

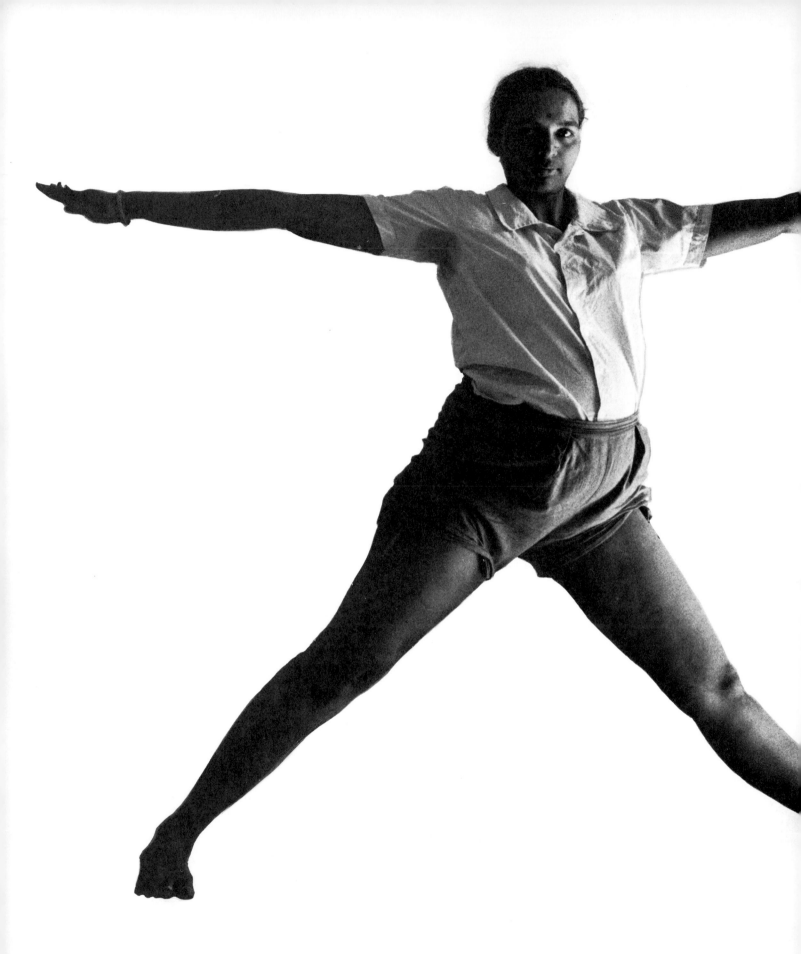

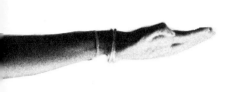

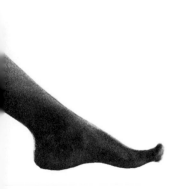

uttihita pārśvakoṇāsana

This powerful Āsana you may perform until the very end of pregnancy.

And your condition brings no limitation or changes.

On the next two pages, don't fail to notice the position of the *feet*.

Feel the *stretching out* from the tips of the fingers to the heel.

And also that the *left leg* and *left arm* are strictly *perpendicular* to the ground.

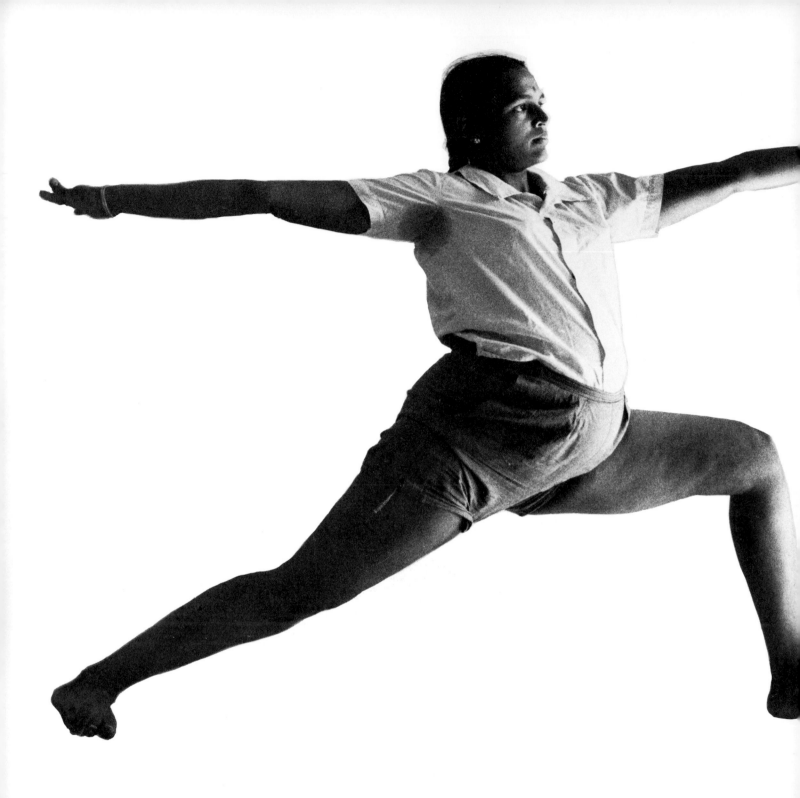

84

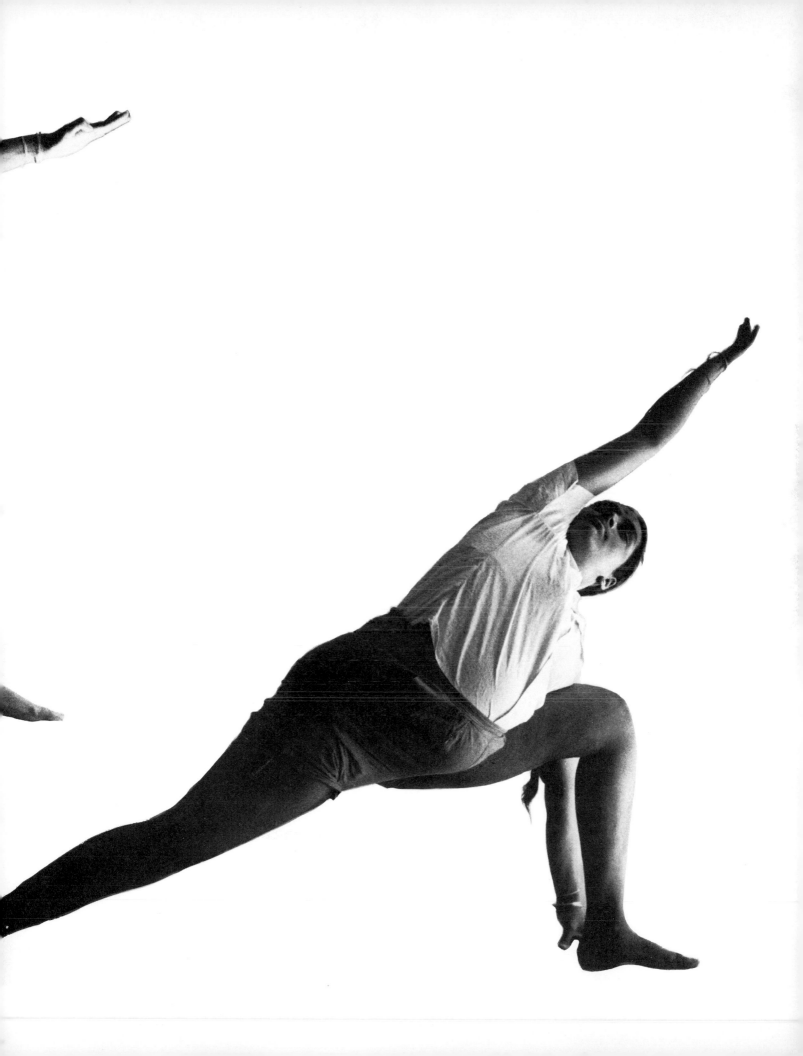

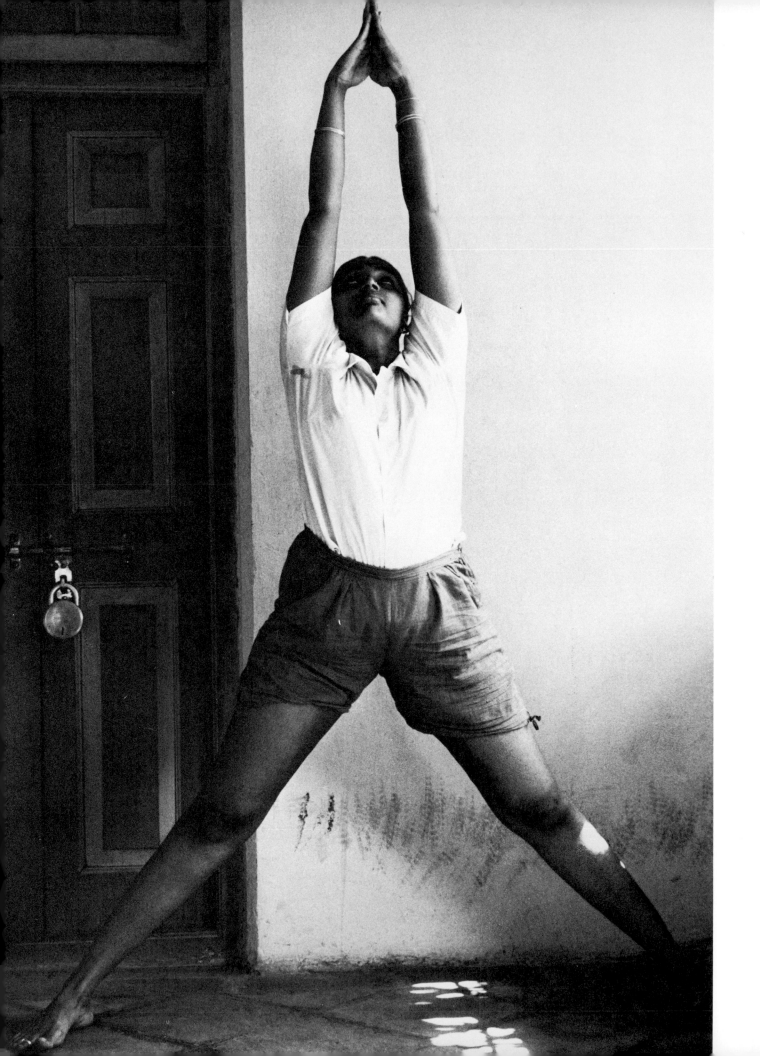

vīrabhadrāsana

Here, again, no limitation due to pregnancy.

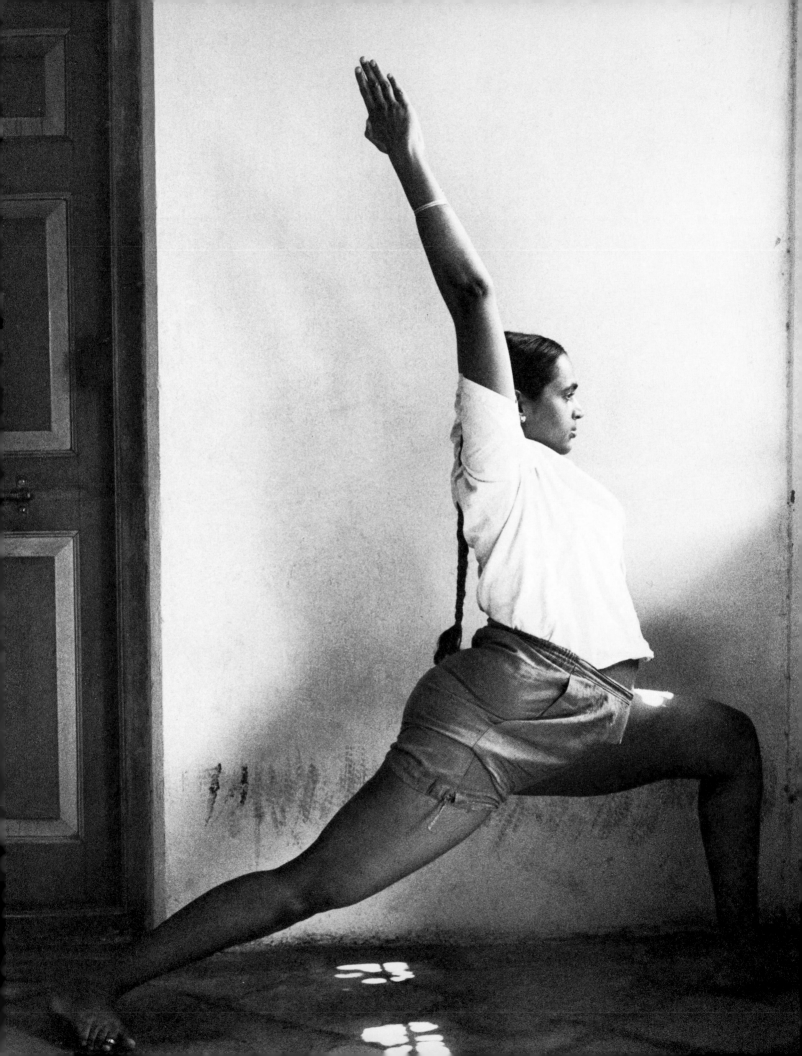

Note carefully that what brings you from starting posture (p. 86) to
full posture (left)
is, simply, the rotation of the feet.
This is where the movement starts.
And it is merely a rotation of the *heels*.
Who carries you? *You?* Or your feet?

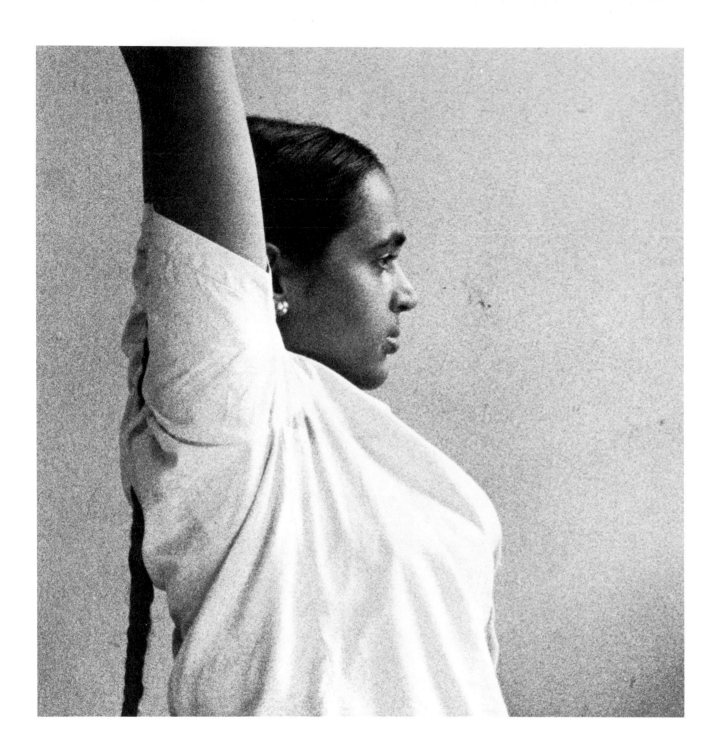

Although the posture is so powerful,
the face remains absolutely quiet;
not the slightest tension.
The face is the mirror of the body.
Indeed, you can read a person from her face.
And since Vanita's body is totally free from tension,
the face cannot but be absolutely peaceful.

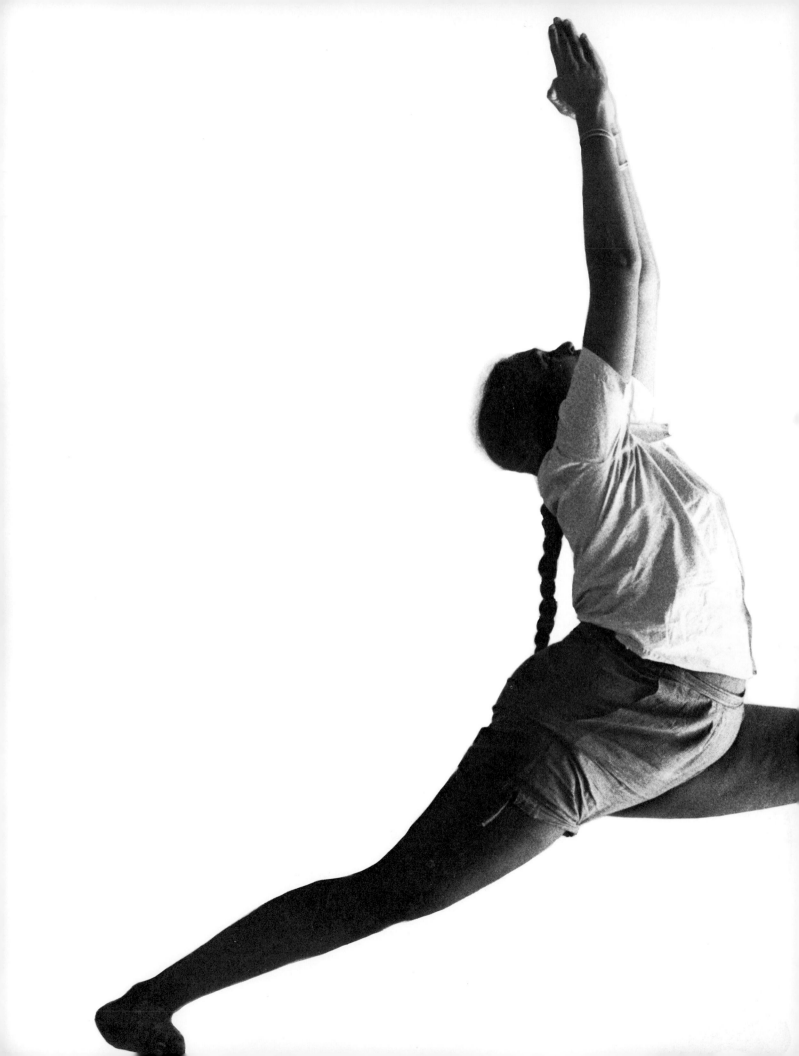

Without moving an inch,
go!
The eyes, only, have been moving *upward*,
going where the hands go . . .
And then, of course, the head follows.

When you *inhale,* open!
And move your hands
as if to touch the sky!

When you *exhale*,
move *forward*,
pushing firmly on the right foot and left knee.

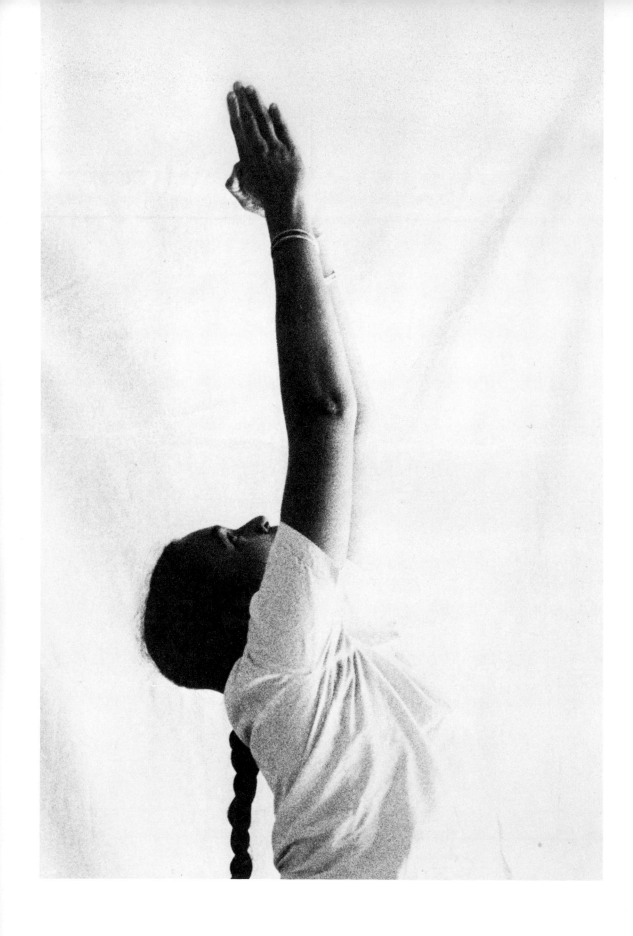

Is it welling
up from below?
Is it dawning
down from above?

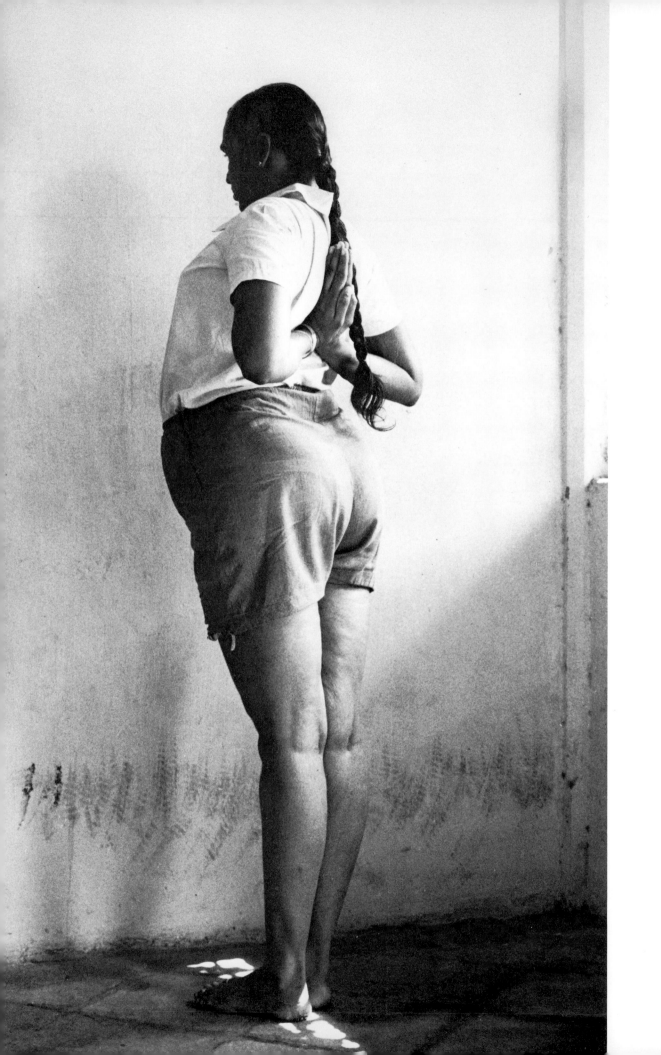

pārśvottānāsana

Here is an Āsana which you are to do only *partly*.

Normally, one goes from backward bending to forward bending, bringing the forehead to touch the knee.

Obviously, even at the beginning of pregnancy, you are to limit forward bending and *never attempt* to make forehead and knee touch.

Be satisfied to make the body horizontal.

First, join your hands *along your back.*

Press them *firmly* one against the other.

The pressure *must be strong*, especially along the outer (little-finger) side of the hands.

While pressing your hands one against the other, push them *up,* along the back, and try to bring them as high as you can.

This is painful in the beginning. This is not easy. But this is the secret, the key to this Āsana.

Unless you keep pressing hard on your hands and bear with the pain, nothing will succeed.

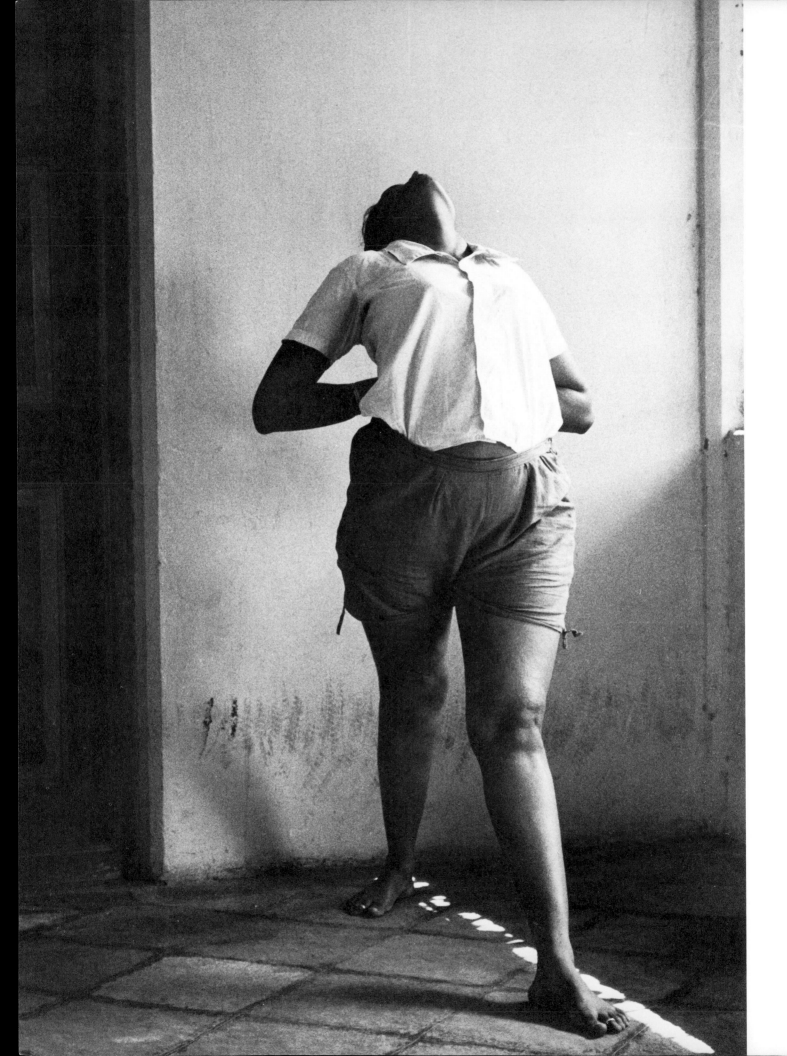

As in the previous Āsana, open your legs, forming a perfect triangle.

Then, again using your *heels* as an axis, rotate your feet, keeping them on one line.

Then, while you *inhale,* with the weight of the body mostly on the rear foot,

bend backward.

The chest opens.

Feel the space between the rib cage and the top of your abdomen.

And, *stretching out,* try to make that space as wide as you can.

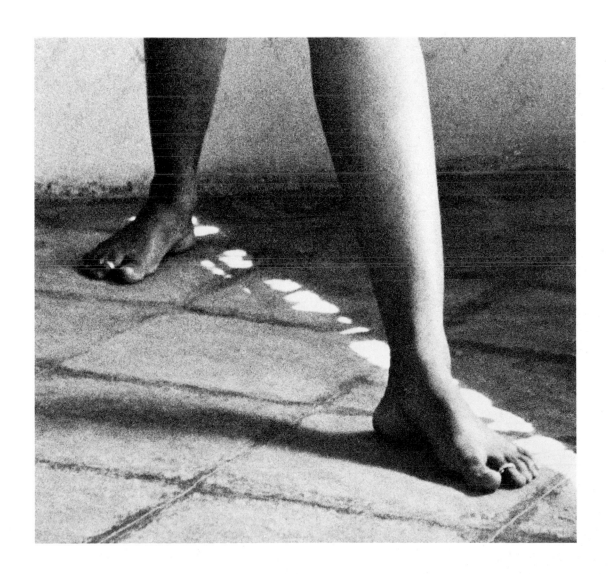

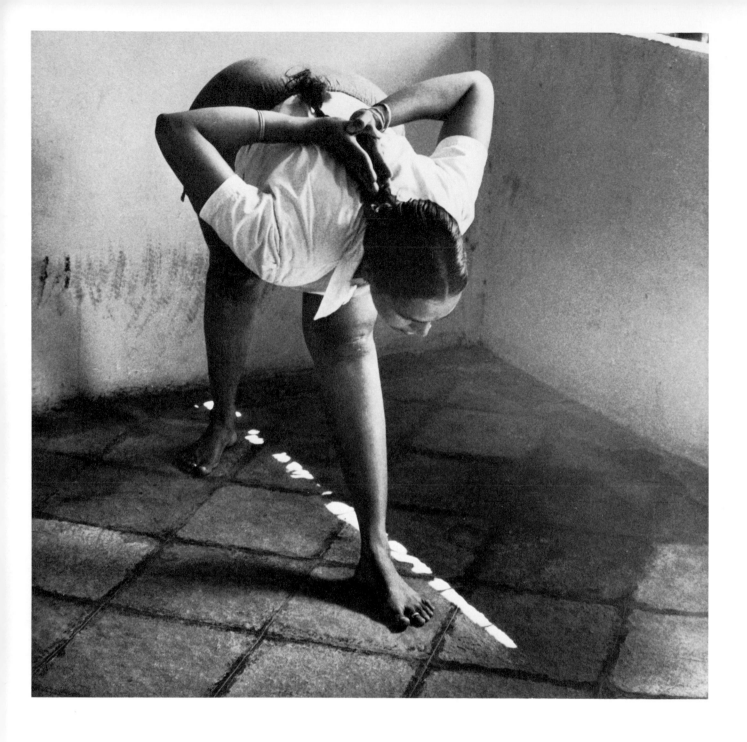

While *exhaling*, shift the weight of your body from your *rear* to your *front* foot.

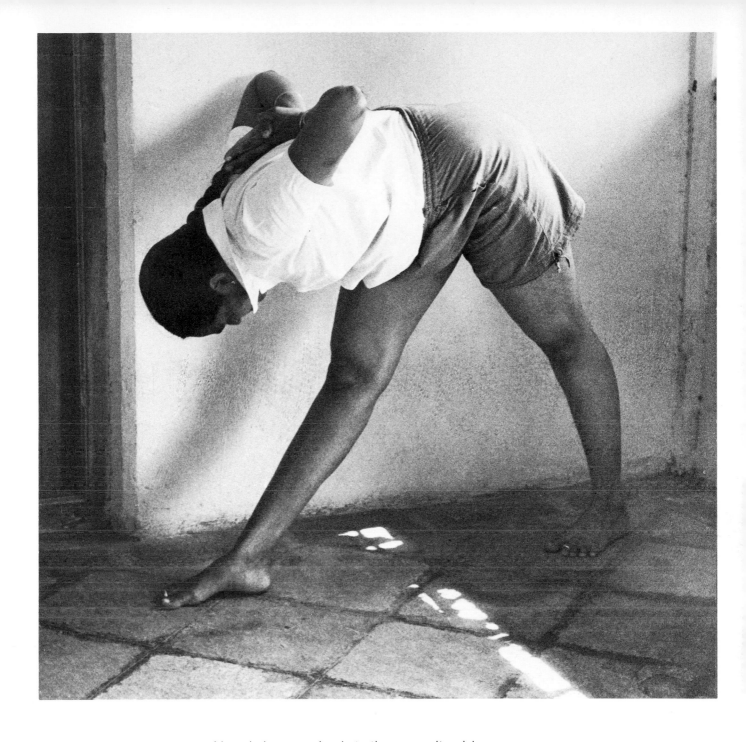

Now, bring your body to the opposite side,
    moving only your *feet*,
    rotating on your *heels*,
    keeping your hands high on your back.
    The strain is terrible.
    Yet there ought to be a deep feeling of acceptance, even of
reverence.

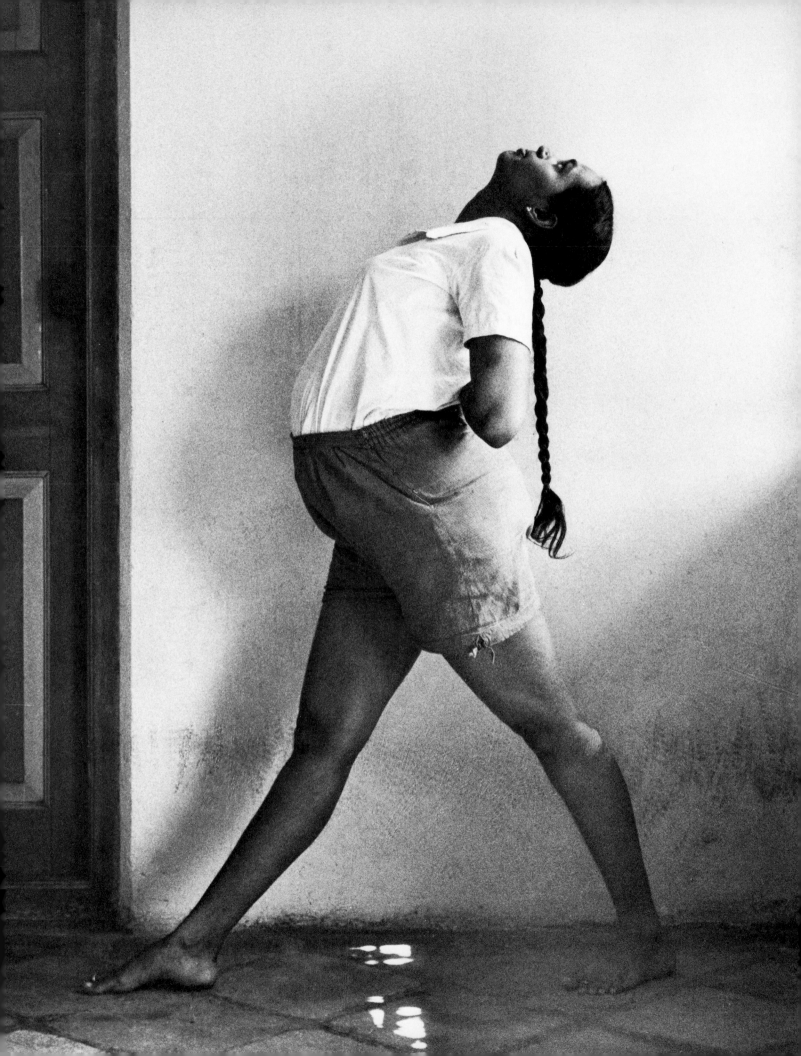

And then, slowly, while inhaling,
    come up.
    Keep pressing hard on your hands!
    And feel the spontaneous deep breathing that starts and
opens your chest.

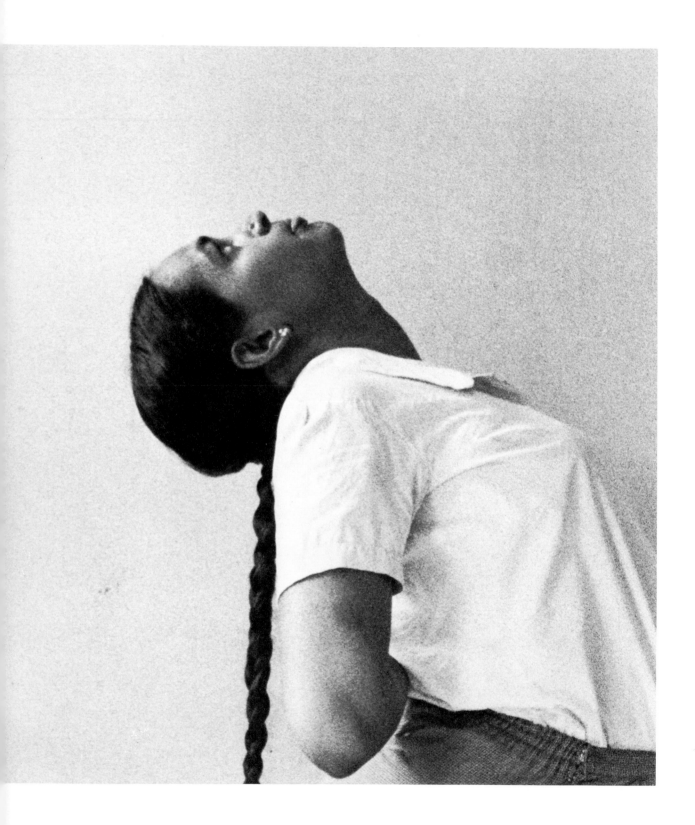

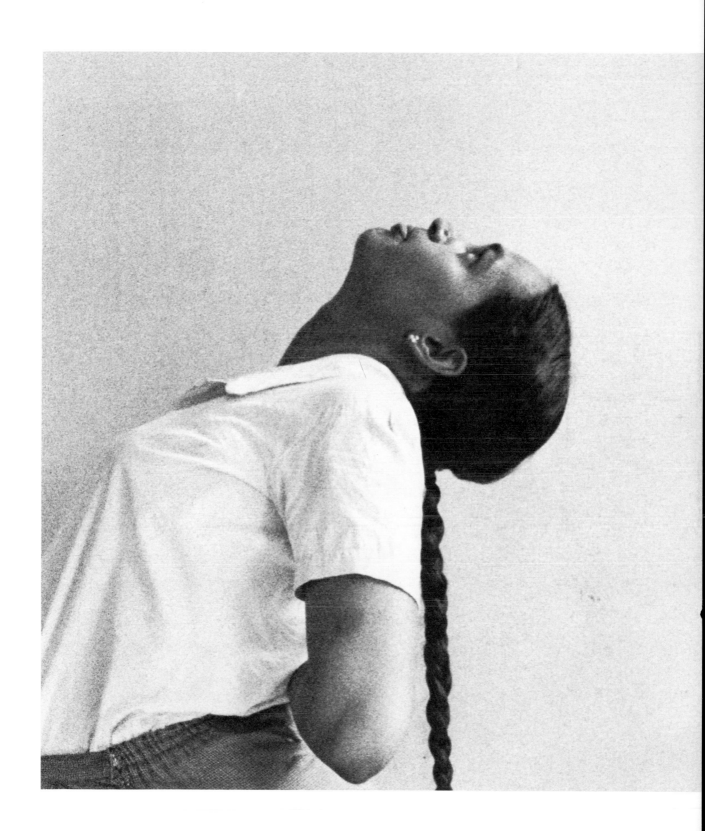

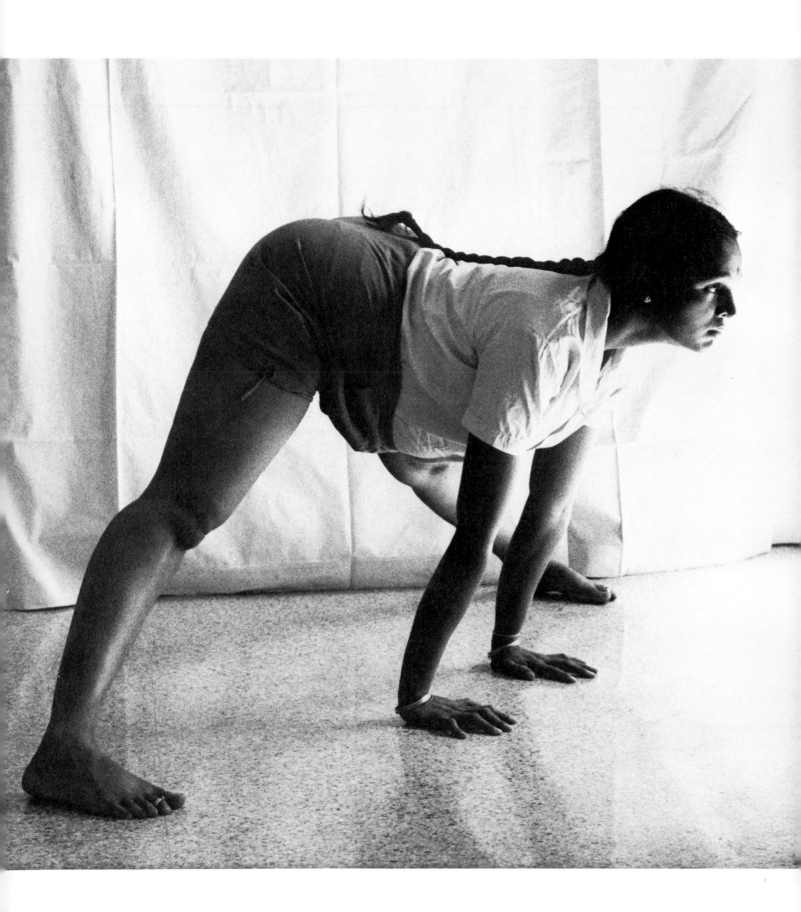

prasārita pādottānāsana

Here, again, some limitations.

Normally, once your hands are on the ground, you bend forward and bring the top of the head down to touch the ground.

This you are *not to do*.

No bending forward at all, at any stage of pregnancy!

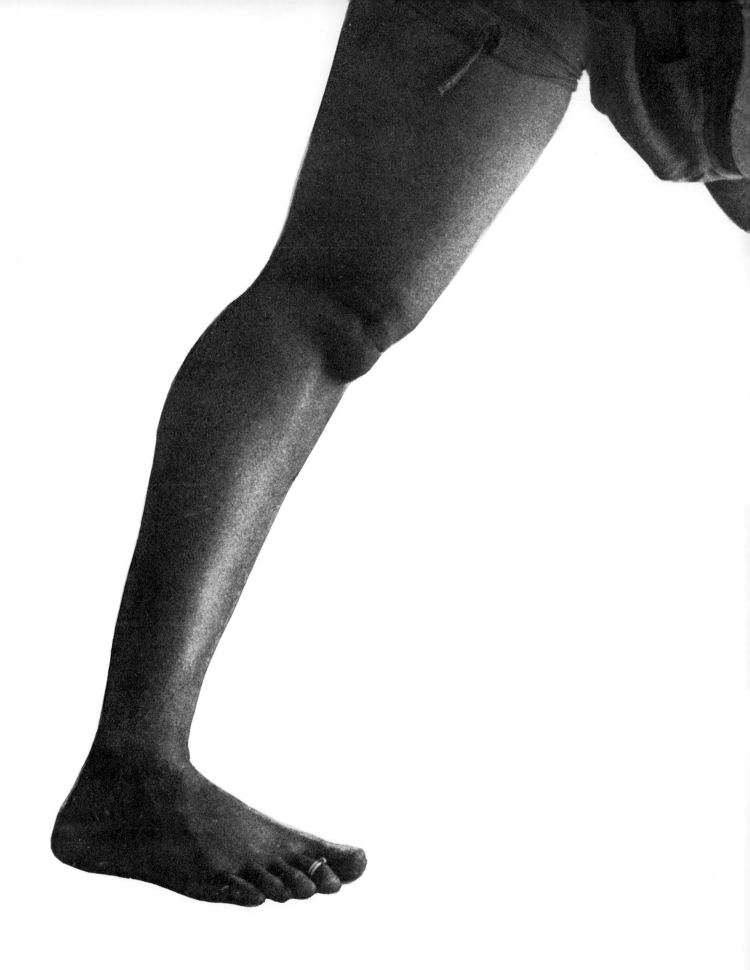

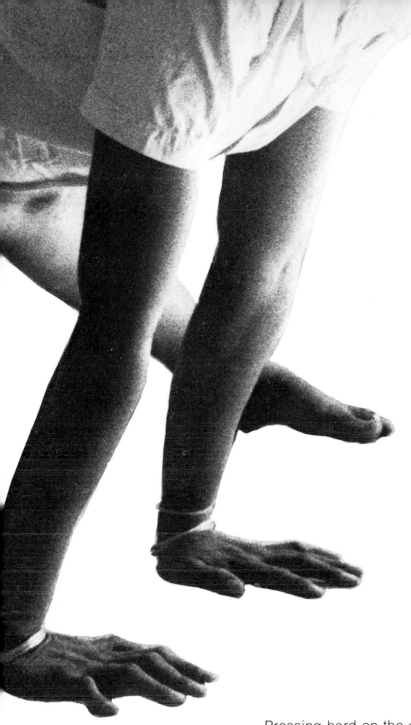

Pressing hard on the ground, with most of your body's weight on your *hands,*

    push sideways on the outer side of your feet.

    At the same time, push *backward* on your hands,

    as if to move your body *forward*.

    And *raise your head!*

    Ah, the tiger may not be very far away!

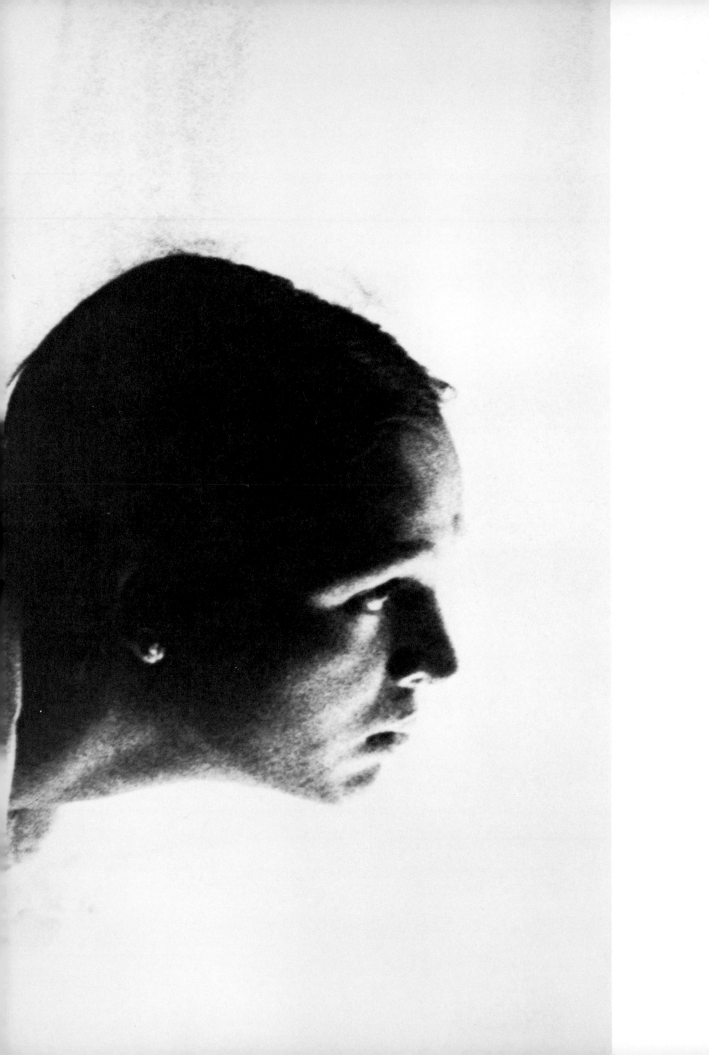

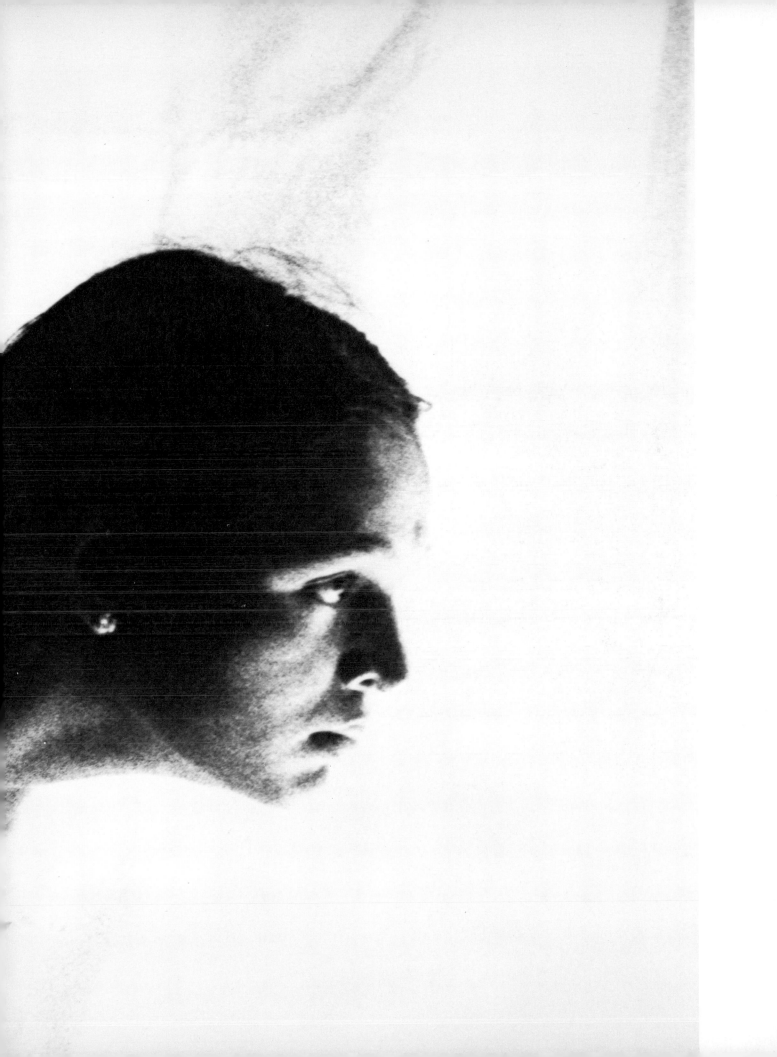

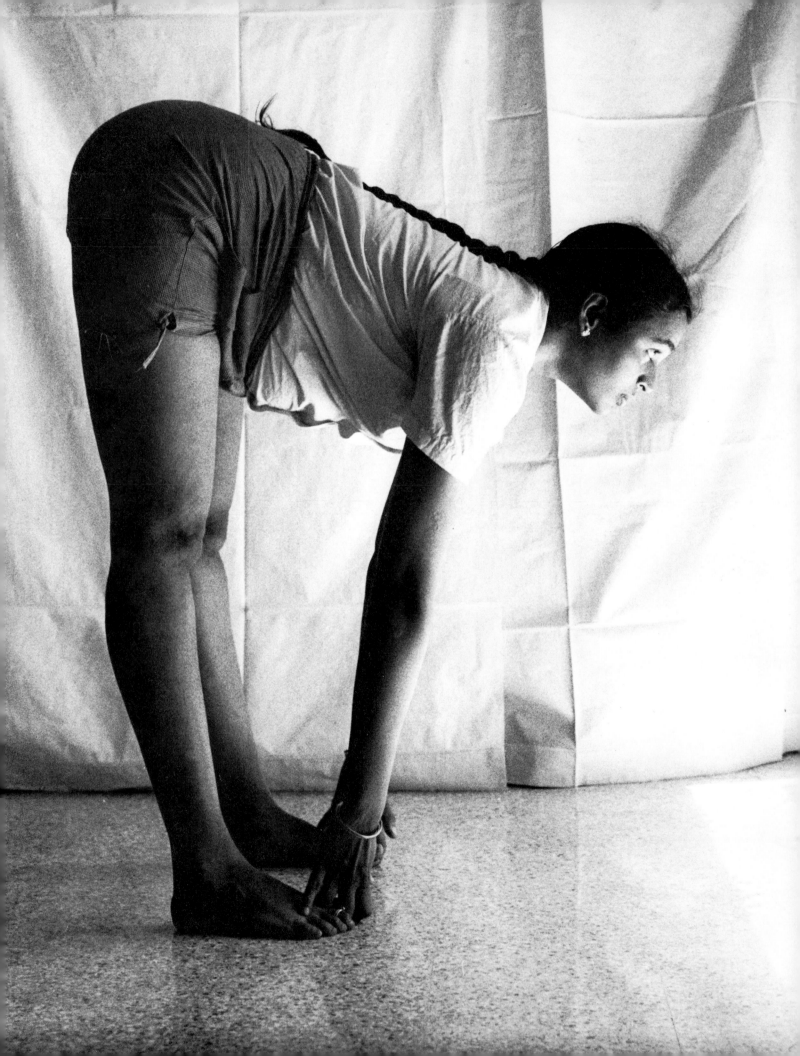

pādāṅguṣṭhāsana

This is very much like a Japanese salutation.

Bend forward
keeping shoulders fully relaxed,
allow the hands to go down *passively*.

You need not touch your feet.
Better if you do, of course,
but what is important is that,
as in the previous Āsana,
you feel a certain point *open*
in your back, between your shoulder blades.

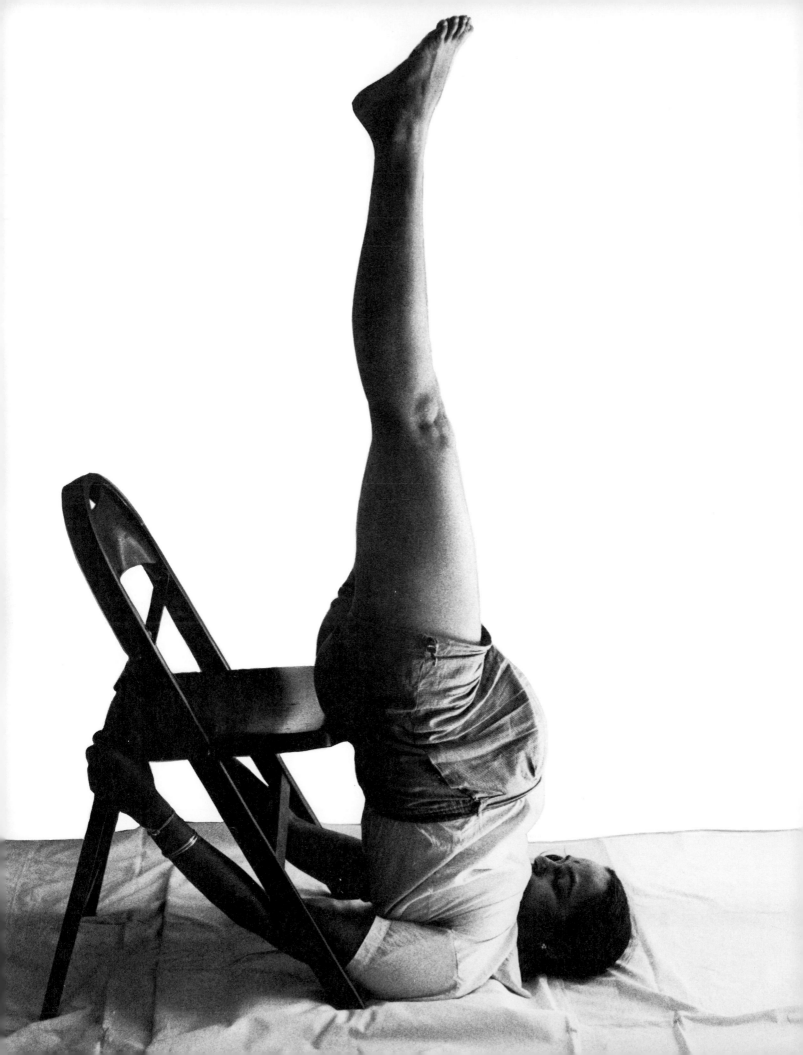

sarvāngāsana

Now comes this other beautiful, most important Āsana.

Since its effects are so profound, let us see it somewhat in detail.

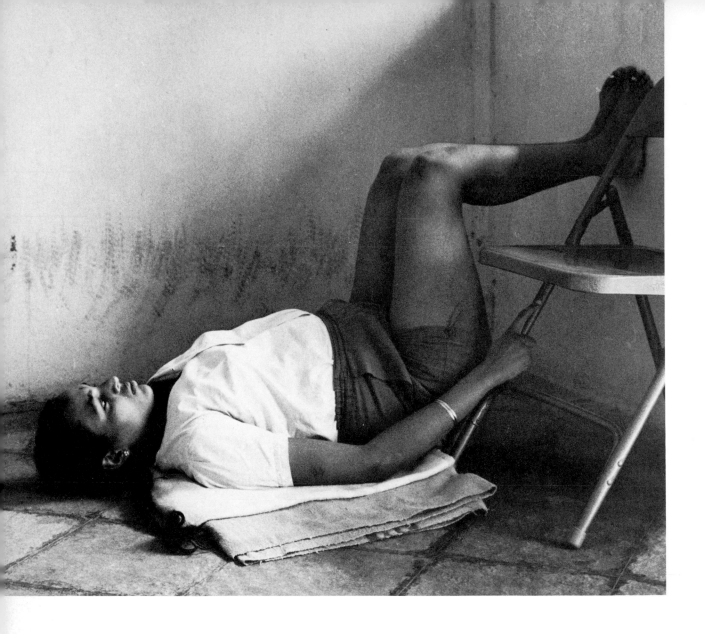

going up

Contrary to what you did for Śīrṣāsana, the head posture, since you are expecting a baby,

    you are to use some external help in order to reach this posture.

    Although you are still *doing it by yourself.*

    You are to *climb on the wall*, as it were, with the use of a chair.

    And keep another chair nearby, which you will be using later on.

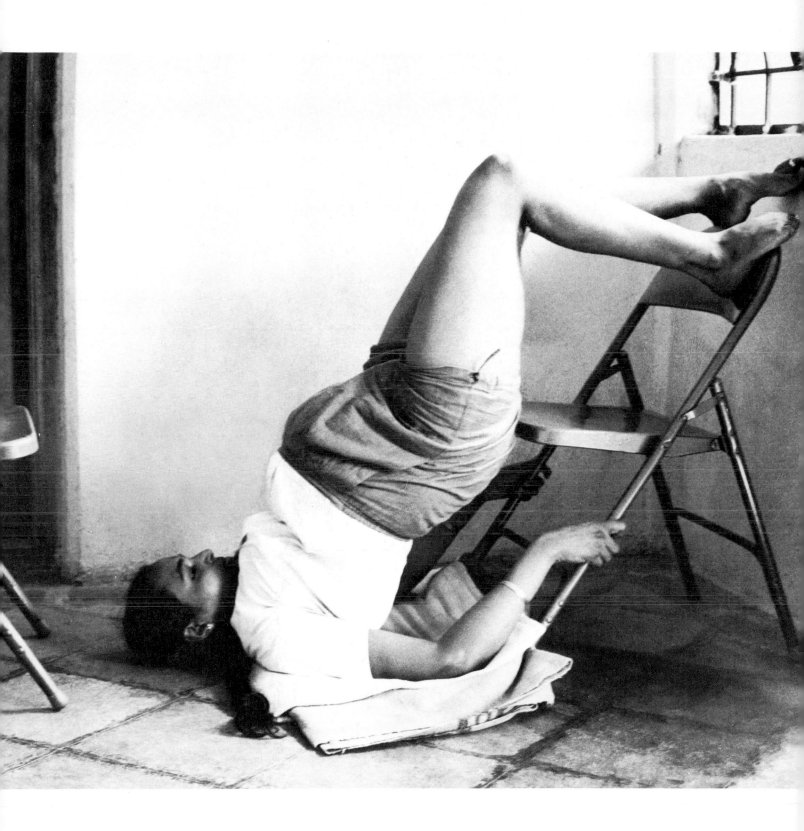

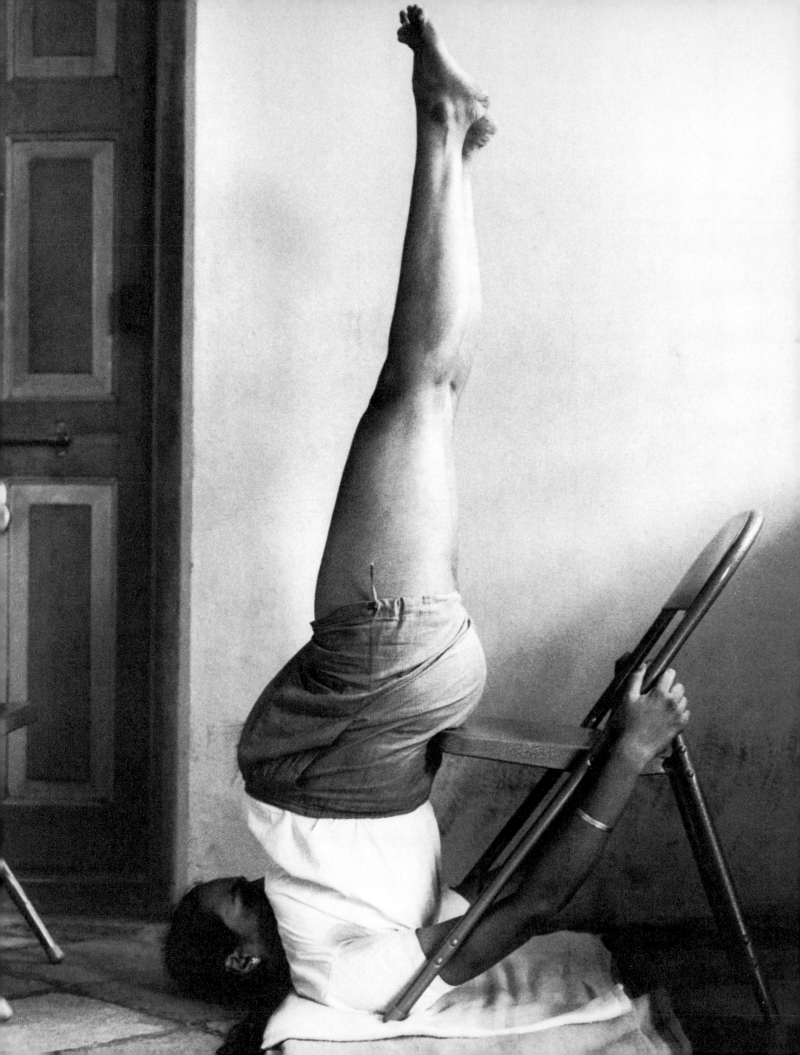

being there

Once you have reached there, once you have taken the posture, you have to adjust with great care.

Pull the chair to yourself and get your arms *within* the legs of the chair.

Then, grabbing the chair firmly, push it against your back. And thus little by little bring your body to rest on your *shoulders,* absolutely *perpendicular* to the ground.

Unless the body is brought to perfect verticality there will be strain and you cannot enjoy lightness and freedom.

Perfect foundation and straightness! Once again!

The secret of this Āsana is in the neck and shoulders.

And *completely let go!*

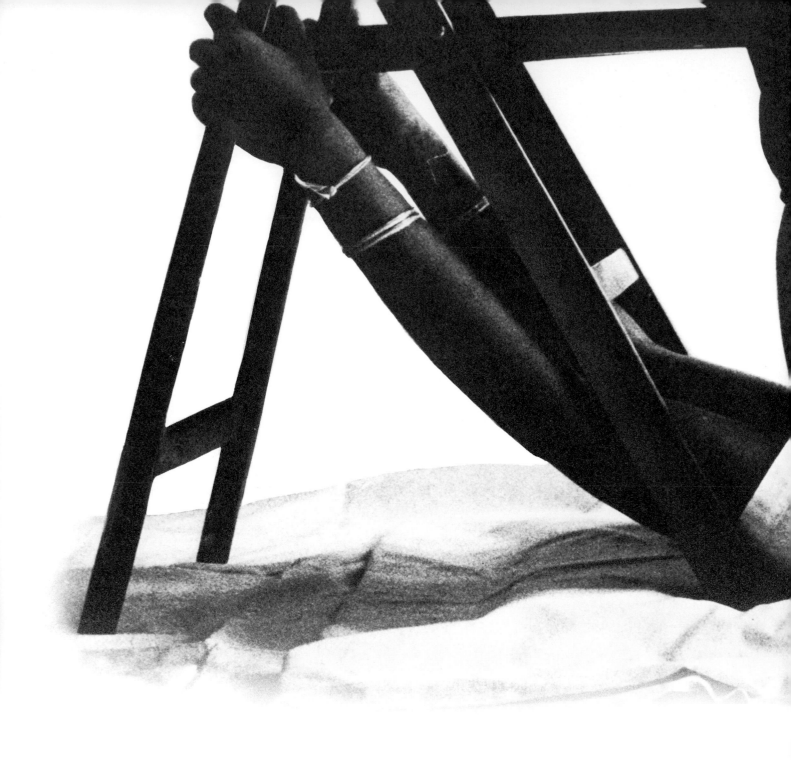

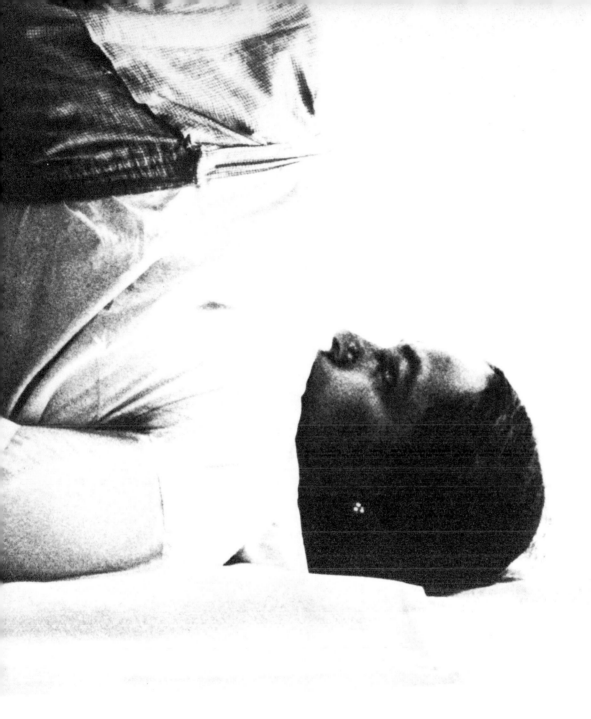

Nowhere is the neck bent so completely.
This proud neck . . .
Ninety degrees. Right angle.
Eighty-eight, eighty-nine will not do.
Complete, unconditional surrender.
But then . . .

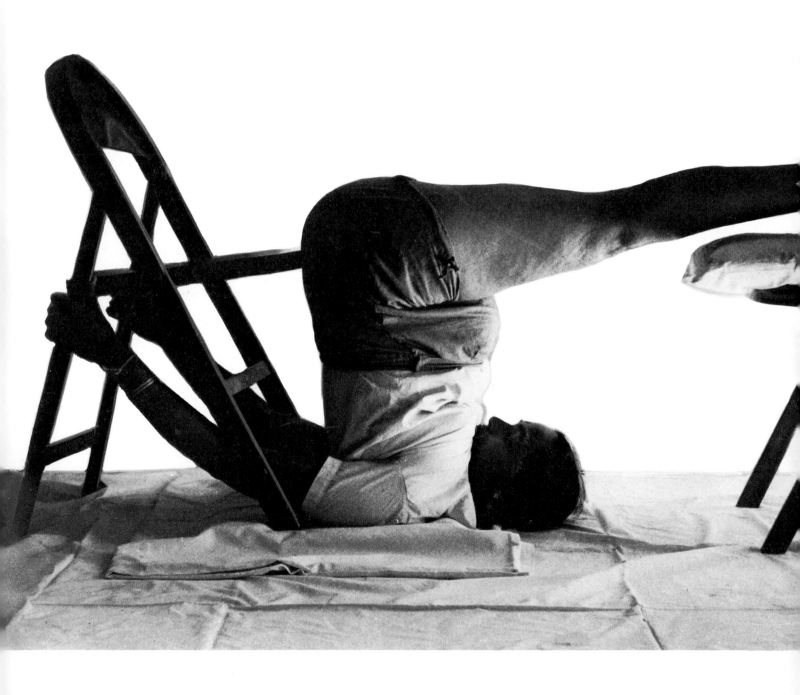

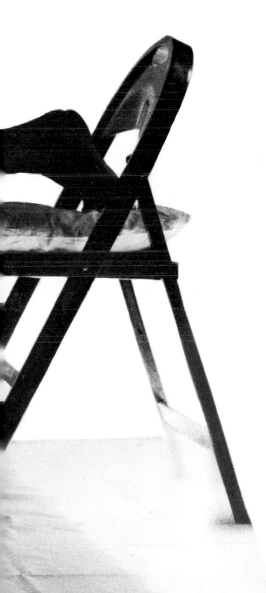

coming back

Were you not pregnant, you would next bring your legs over your head and, keeping your trunk perpendicular to the ground, bring your feet to touch the ground way back behind your head.

The purpose being to bring deeper relaxation to your neck and shoulders.

But owing to your present condition, this *you are absolutely not to do.*

Use the other chair, which you have kept nearby. Draw it to you and bring your feet to rest on it.

You have put a pillow on it, which makes it all even more comfortable and restful.

Remember . . .

"The posture ought to be pleasant and easy!"

Whenever you feel tired or upset or a little depressed,

take this posture for *five* or *ten* minutes.

Nothing to do. Just let go.

Within a few minutes you will be surprised to feel that, all tensions gone, you begin to enjoy a deep, effortless, mysterious rest and peace.

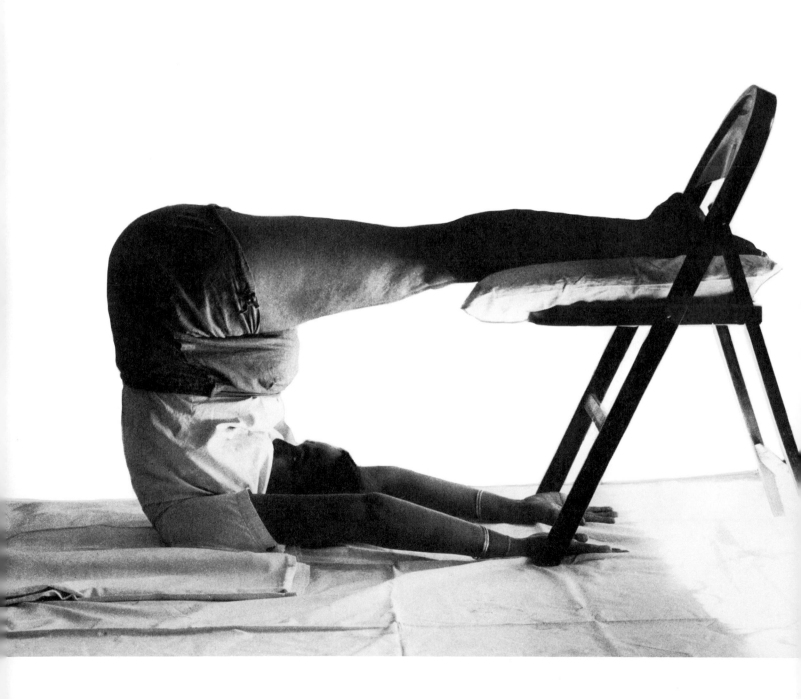

halāsana

Actually, on your way, you have met this other Āsana, Halāsana.

You have disentangled your arms from the first chair, of course, in order to move the second chair.

Now you stretch your arms *behind* your head.

Trunk is still perfectly perpendicular to the ground.

Arms and legs are parallel to each other and parallel to the ground. And strictly perpendicular to the trunk of the body.

Right angles everywhere.

But no strain.

Feel the deep relaxation, the complete freedom in the neck and shoulders and the *spontaneous,* full breathing *in your back.*

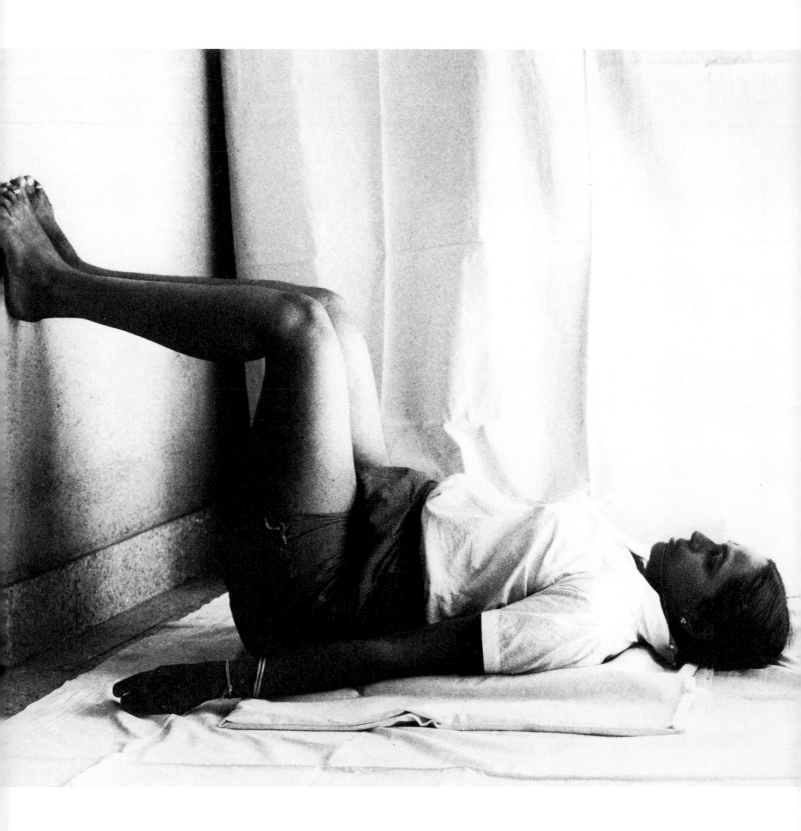

coming back

Once you have fully enjoyed Halāsana, you may come back for
good.

Bring your arms forward and, with your fingers, press hard on
the ground.

This pressure of hands and fingers slows down your descent.

As much as you can, let your back get in touch with the
ground *one vertebra* after another.

And then, keeping your feet on the wall, *rest.*

The fact that your feet are against the wall, keeping your
thighs at *right angles* with the body, gives complete relaxation to
your back and *pelvis.*

And, indeed, this shows on your face . . .

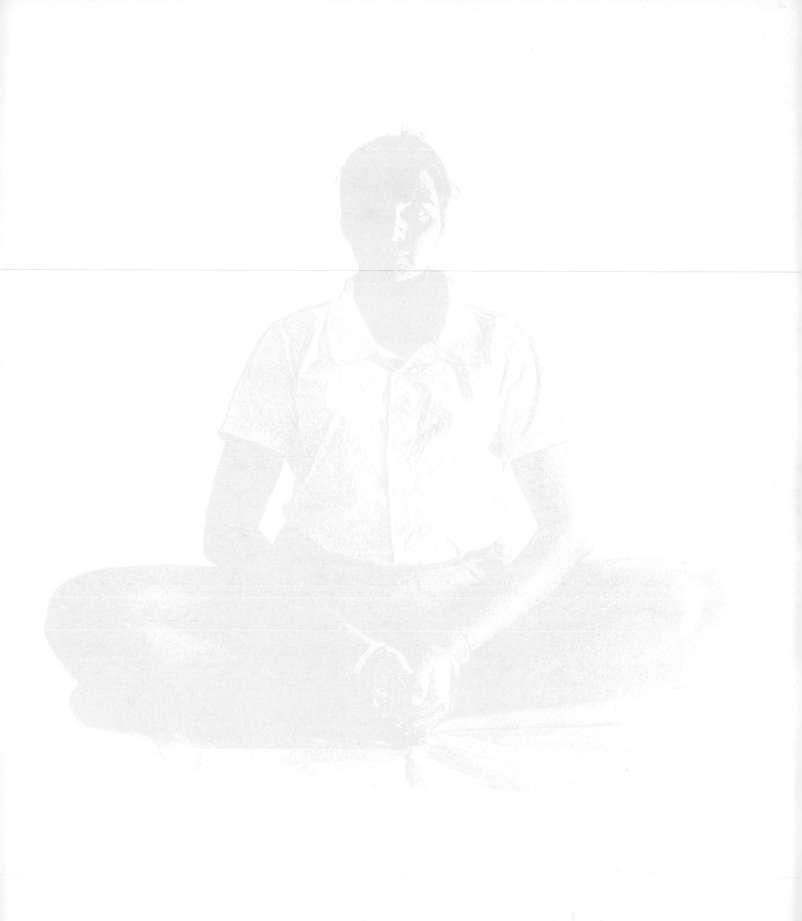

the sitting postures

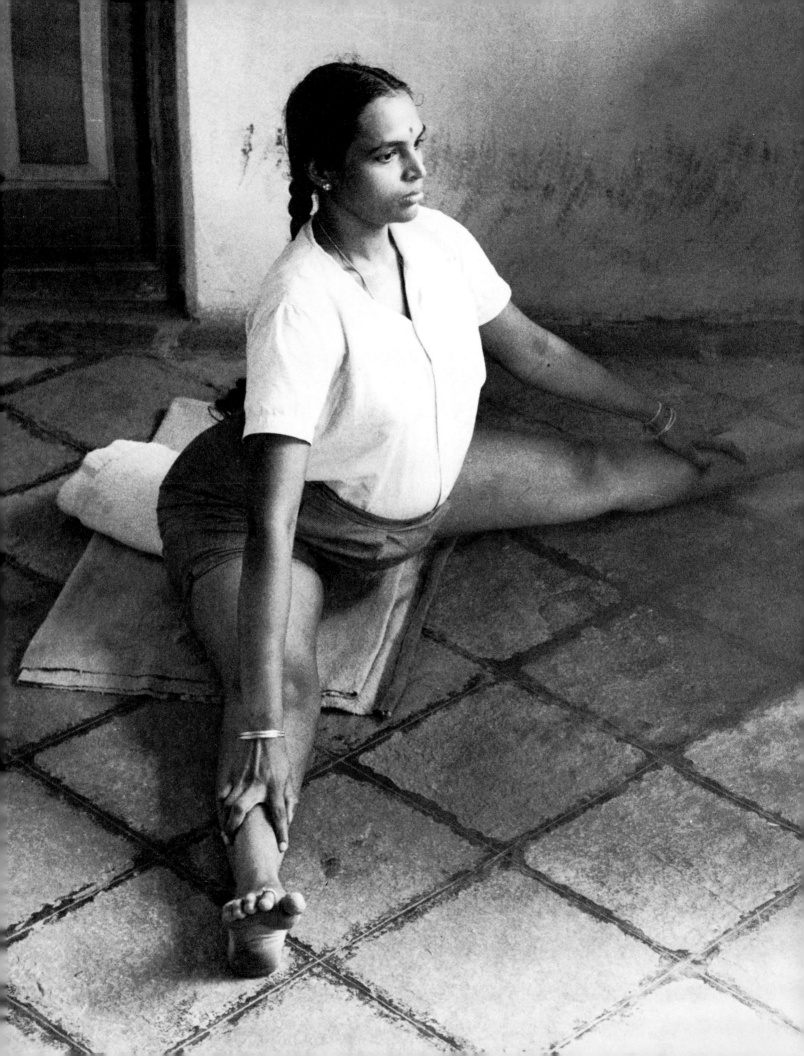

upaviṣṭha koṇāsana

In this Āsana, after sitting with your legs open at right angles—
ninety degrees again!—you would bend forward and bring your
forehead down to touch the ground.

Owing to your condition, this, of course, you are *not to do*.

Be satisfied to achieve *perfect sitting*.

A rare yet simple achievement.

Keep your legs at right angles with knees fully relaxed.

Keep shoulders relaxed as well, so that your hands come to
rest lightly, weightlessly, on your legs.

And then, every time you *inhale*, raise your head and bring
your big stomach slightly *forward* as if to let it rest, ultimately, on
the ground.

And feel how the back is opening, breathing again, *spontaneous* and deep.

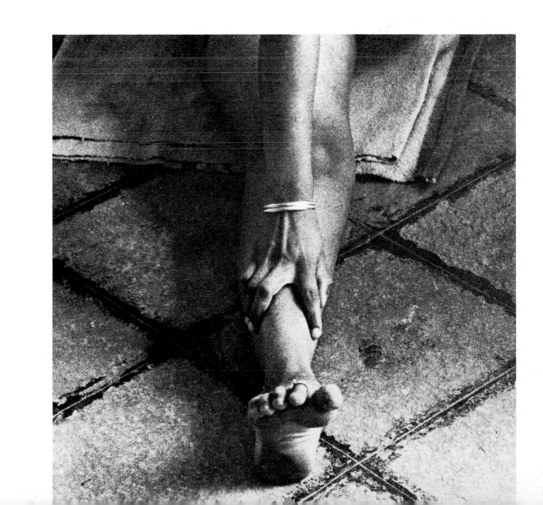

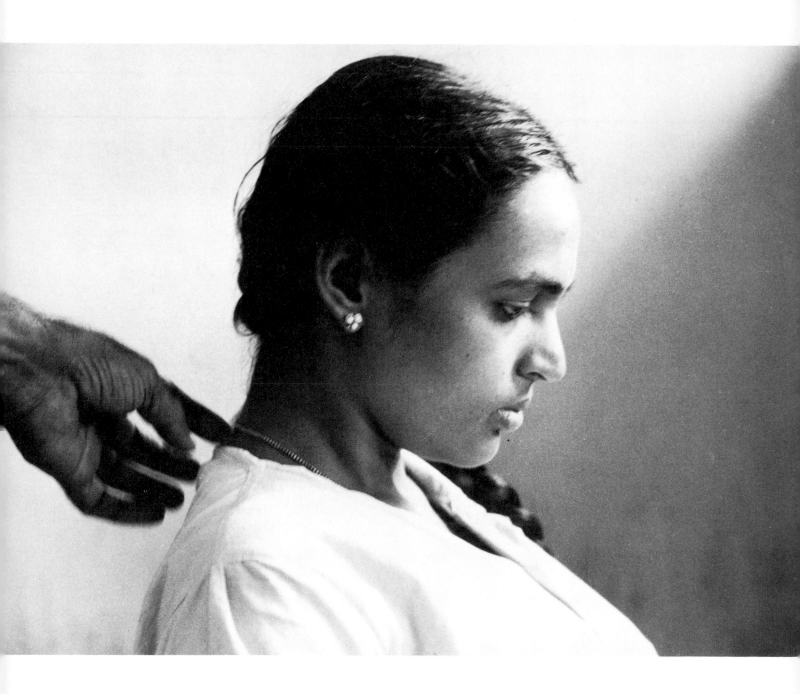

This neck!

Just as, by gently turning the pegs,
one tunes a Stradivarius
did you know that by merely moving the neck
you tune the entire body?

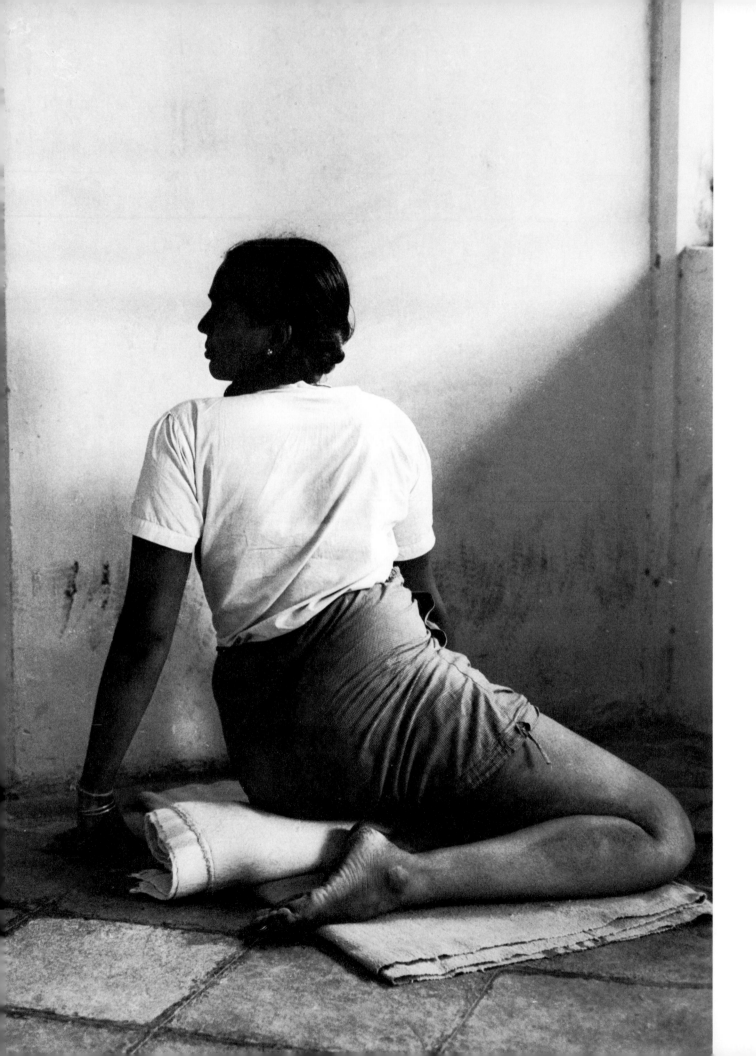

bharadvājāsana

With a good deal of bending back and forth, your back has been warming up.

But the spine works *around* its axis as much as, if not more than, bending forward and backward.

Torsion is basic to its functioning.

And without this ability, this *twisting* faculty . . . you could not be born.

In order to progress along the birth canal, these torsions are absolutely necessary.

Bharadvājāsana will make you enjoy this torsion.

In order to make things more comfortable and easy, you may use a folded blanket and rest *one buttock* on it, as you see in the picture.

But if the Āsana is understood properly, this may not be necessary.

And, indeed, there has been much misunderstanding about this posture.

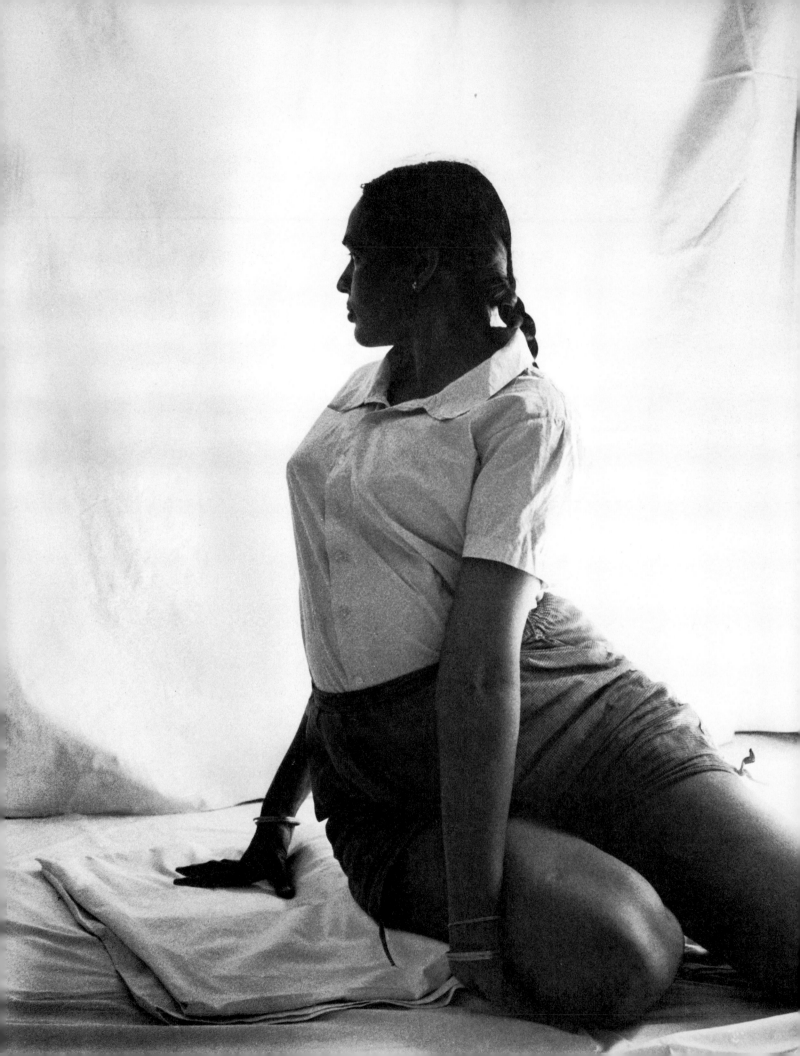

Since in this Āsana the weight of the body is ultimately to rest on *your hands,* you are to place these hands very carefully.

Suppose you turn, first, to your right.

Place your *right* hand on the ground, just where it falls naturally.

Fingers are pointing to your right, away from you.

Then place the fingers of your *left* hand under your *right knee.*

Thus your hands are in *opposite* directions:

the fingers of the right hand are pointing to the right, away from your self or the center of your body,

the fingers of your left hand are pointing to your left, toward your self, toward your center.

But both your hands must be on a line, an axis parallel to the south – north axis of your body.

Let us define these axes very clearly.

There are three axes to the human body.

One is vertical as you know now.

There are two more:

One going from your back to your front. Which we might call south – north. if you are simply standing we might say that you are *facing north.* And then, of course, south is at your back.

And the last axis is transverse, which we shall call east – west.

It is the normal axis of your shoulders or your hips.

And as you are *facing north,* east is to your right and west to your left.

All right. In Bharadvājāsana, while your *hips* remain on this transverse, *east – west axis,* your shoulders will move *ninety degrees* to the *south – north axis.*

And it is on this *south – north axis* that you have placed both your hands very carefully.

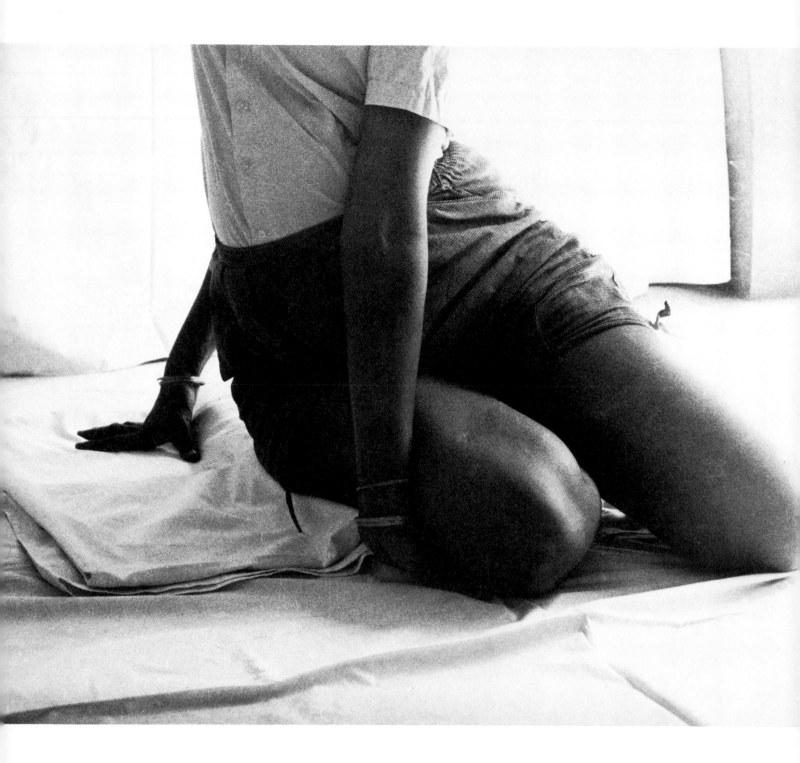

What are you to do in order to bring your shoulders and your head to face *east* — that is to say, to your *right?*

Simply straighten your arms and press gently with both your hands on the ground,

as if to *lift* yourself, as if to raise yourself *on your hands*.

This simple pressure and the *stretching out* of your arms brings you to face *east*.

Together with the *torsion*, your shoulders and your body have been *going up* (you *raised* yourself on your hands),

and you can feel not only the *torsion*, but a kind of very gentle and deeply pleasant *easing up* in the spine.

The whole movement, actually, is not merely a torsion, it is a *spiral!*

Let it be said once again that it ought to be *very gentle;* a twisting, yes, but mostly a *stretching out* which starts in the palms of your hands.

Something you sometimes do — spontaneously, unconsciously — when, hands resting on a balcony on the morning of a very clear day, you feel that life is so young and so fresh, that you are terribly, terribly happy.

Then come back,
simply relaxing the arms, the hands, the shoulders . . .

Then, of course, turn to the other side.

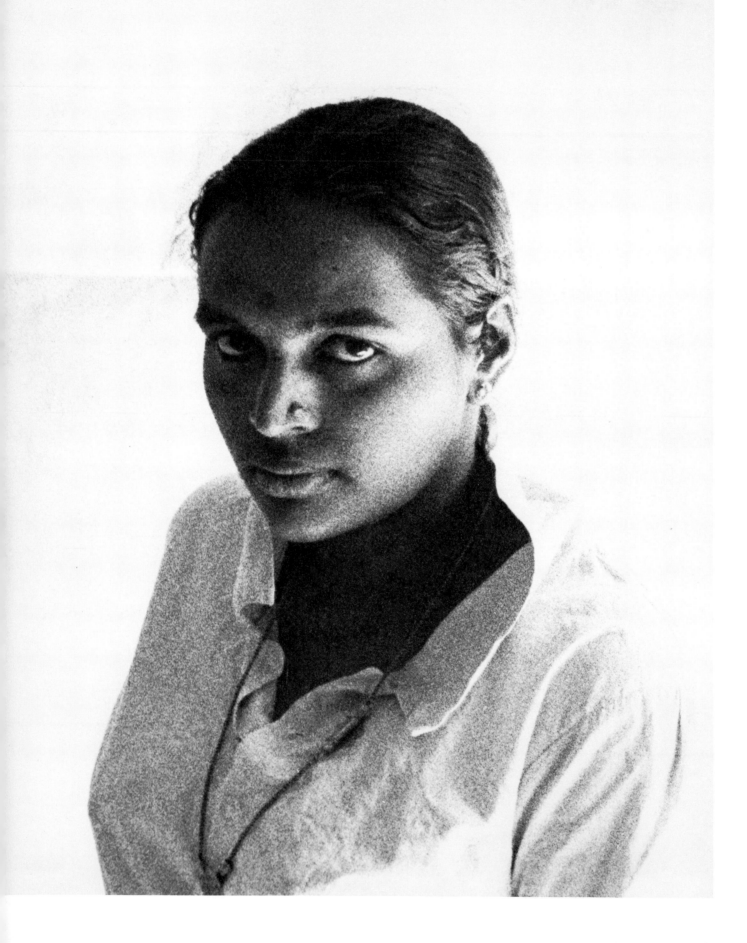

Now
you are getting very near . . .

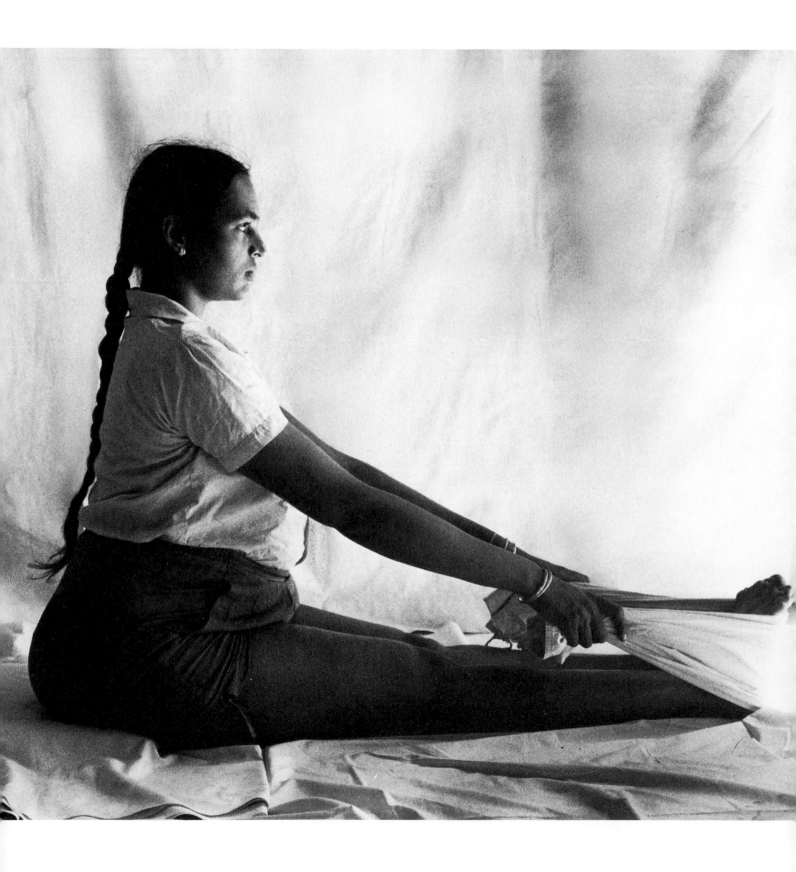

paśchimottānāṣana

The essence of Yoga.

Simplicity itself: bend forward and, *without bending your knees,* touch your forehead to your knees.

Nothing could be more simple.

And, then, of course, more difficult.

Since you are pregnant, you are not to bend forward and neither should you attempt to make your forehead touch your knees.

But, using a simple aid, you may still reap all the fruits of this posture:

take a towel, put it round your feet and keep both ends in your hands.

And then, begin to pull gently.

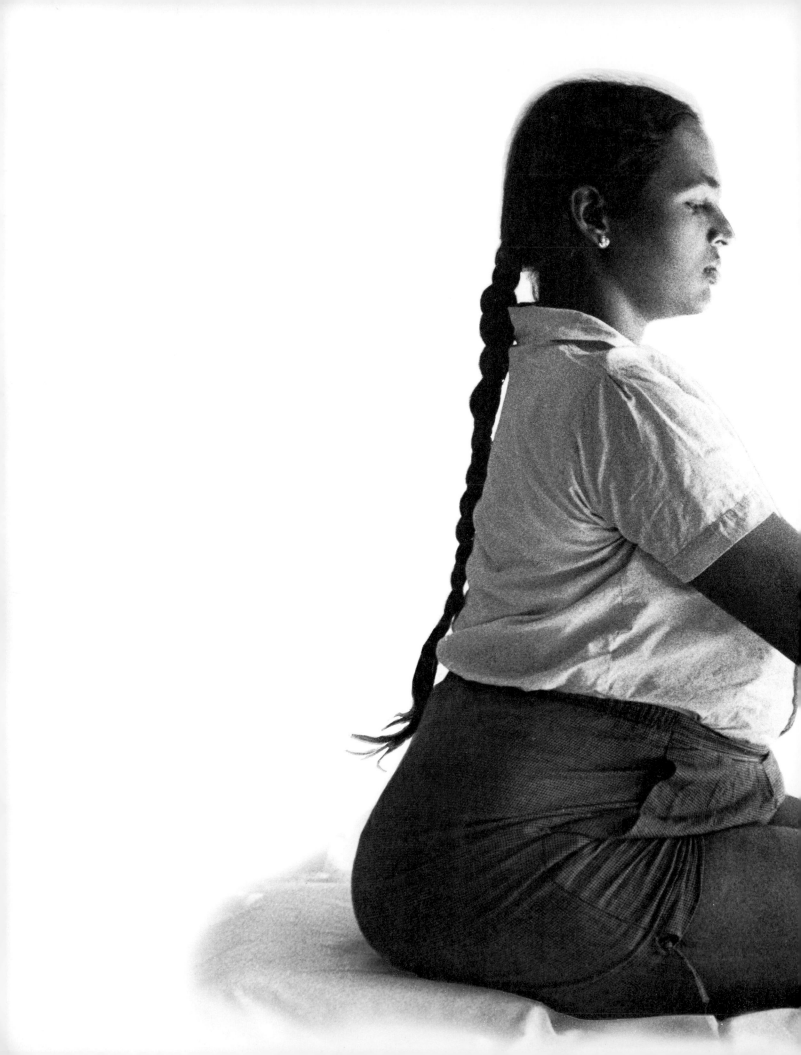

Pulling. Why? In order to bring the trunk forward, of course.

But, the moment you start pulling, the strain in your legs and, mostly, at the back of your knees becomes unbearable.

(The towel ought to go round the *top* of your feet, very close to your *toes,* in order to keep the feet at a *right angle* with the legs.)

There you are, trapped in unavoidable, unescapable contradiction:

pulling brings at the same time

the desirable end — your trunk, indeed, goes forward —

and the pain that stops everything!

What to do?

The secret is *not to react.*

Keep pulling, of course. Don't give up.

But keep pulling so *gently* that you *let go, in the legs,* right where the terrible pain is.

You are with pain. You accept. *You don't fight.*

You progress *inch by inch.*

And, if you *keep pulling* with *legs fully relaxed*

(see how it shows in Vanita),

suddenly deep, spontaneous abdominal breathing starts

and pain vanishes totally.

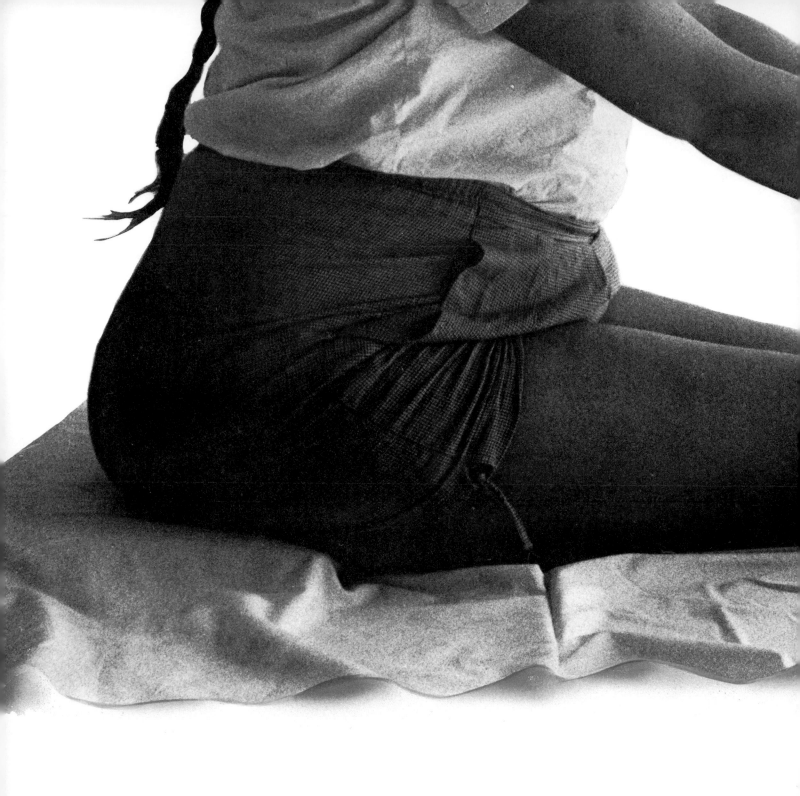

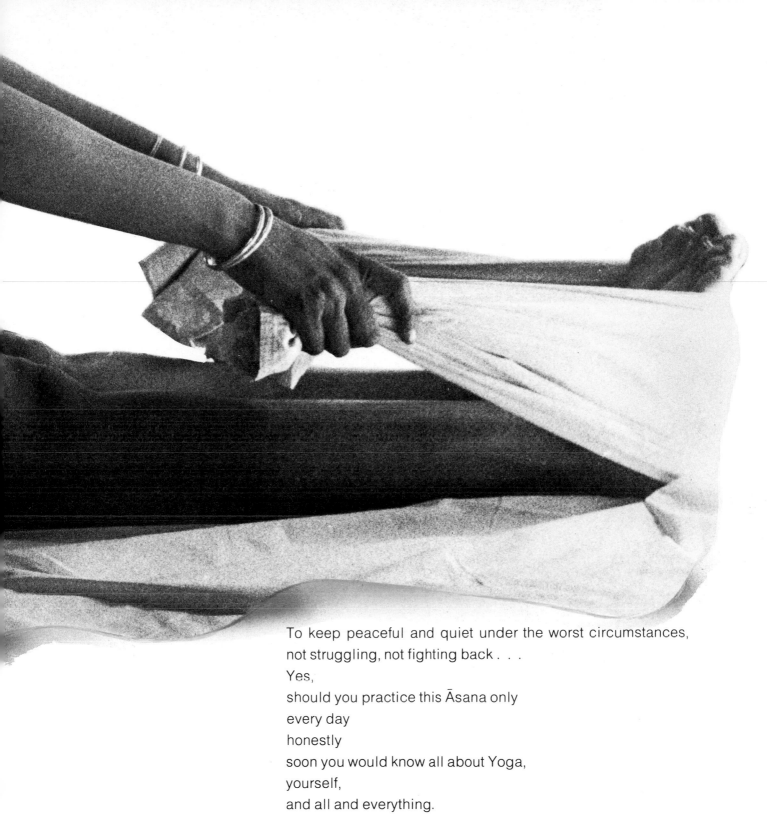

To keep peaceful and quiet under the worst circumstances,
not struggling, not fighting back . . .
Yes,
should you practice this Āsana only
every day
honestly
soon you would know all about Yoga,
yourself,
and all and everything.

Says Lord Krishna:
—Arjuna! Who is the real lord of this chariot of yours?

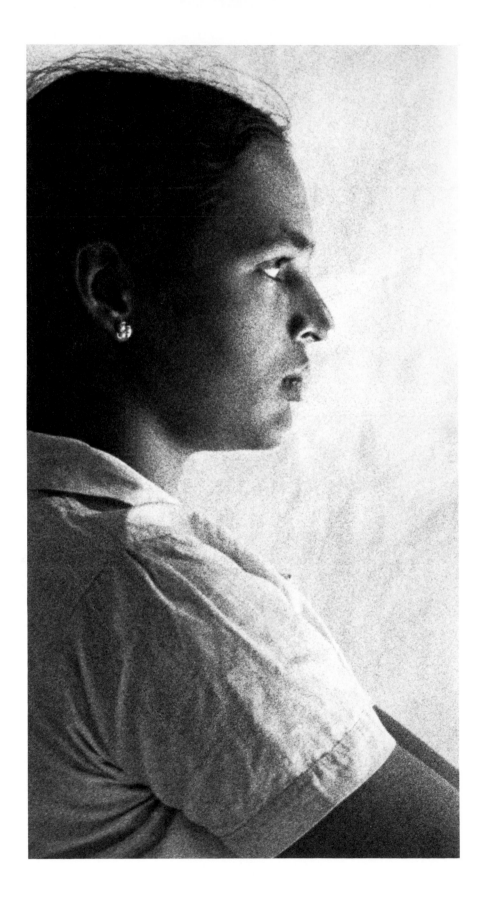

Sageness within,
Kingliness without.

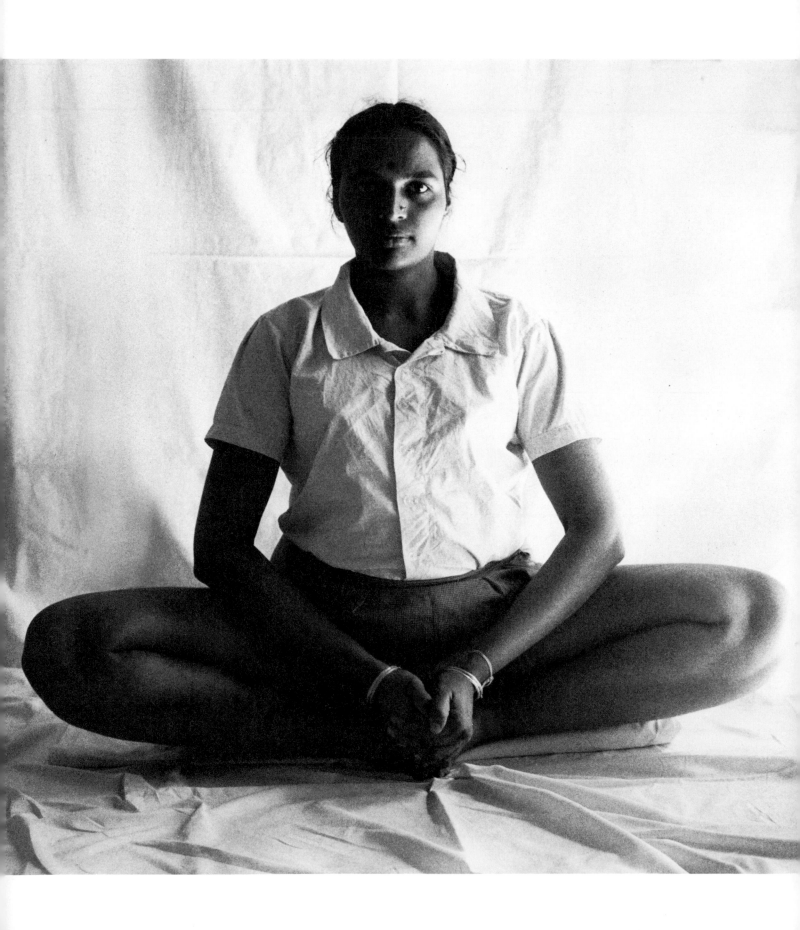

baddha koṇāṣana

We are not far from the end of our session.
>As a conclusion, before you rest,
>here is one last simple Āsana.
>Simple . . .
>And most beneficial for expecting mothers, who may keep practicing it until the very last day.

>Beginners may sit
>on a folded blanket
>and with their backs to a wall,
>which will make things easier in the beginning.

>Open your legs.
>Join your feet *sole to sole.*
>Keep them together with your hands.
>And while you press them one against the other, try to lift the upper part of the feet,
>pulling on your back
>and raising your head.

>That's all.
>With, again, one most important point:
>the head goes *up* each time you *inhale.*
>Then the chest opens
>and deep, *spontaneous abdominal* breathing begins.

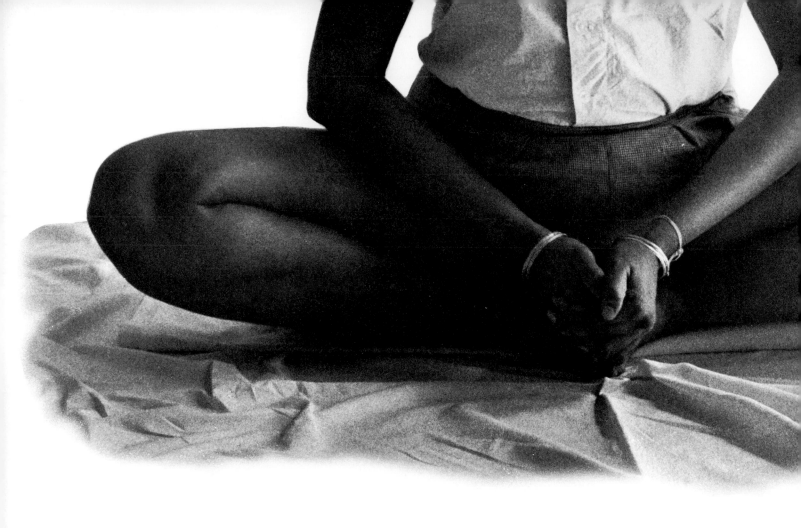

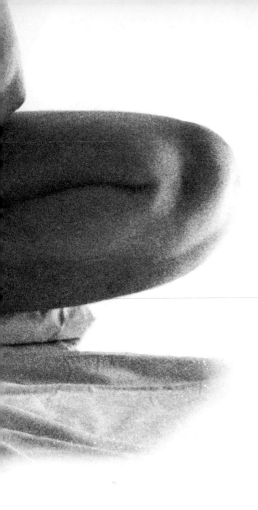

Don't try to bring your knees down forcibly, don't try to *push* them
down. That would not do.

As your chest starts to open and deep breathing begins,
your knees will come down spontaneously, effortlessly.

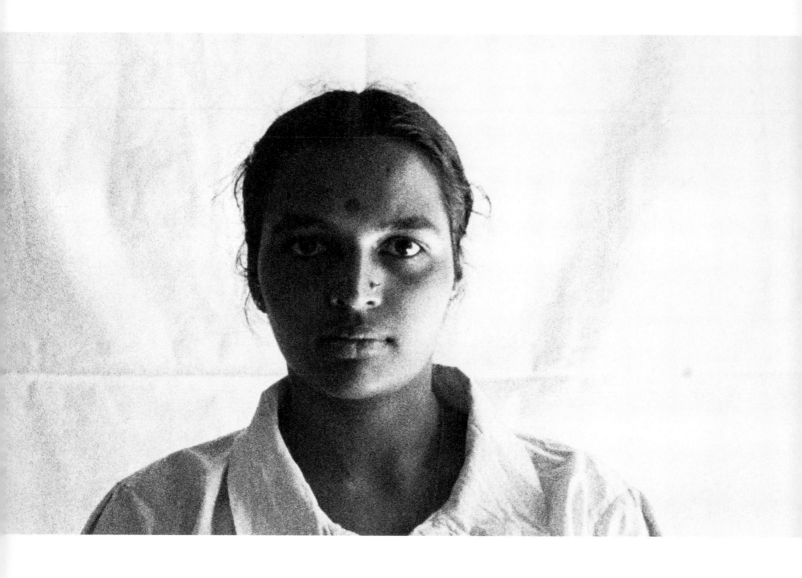

Rejoice.
Your toiling is over.
You are about to reap
the fruits of your courage, of your patience.

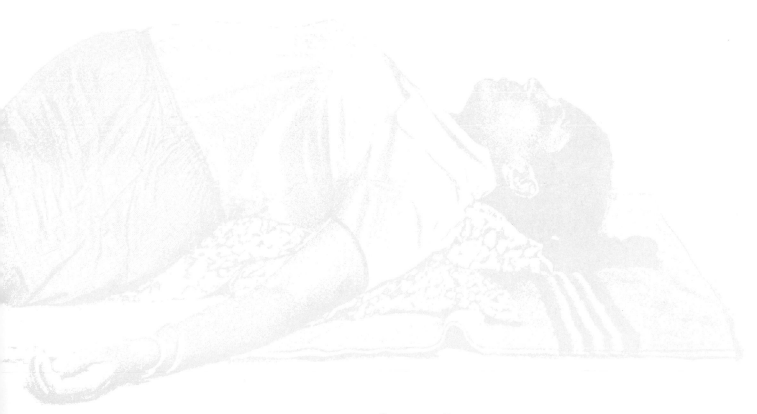

the lying postures

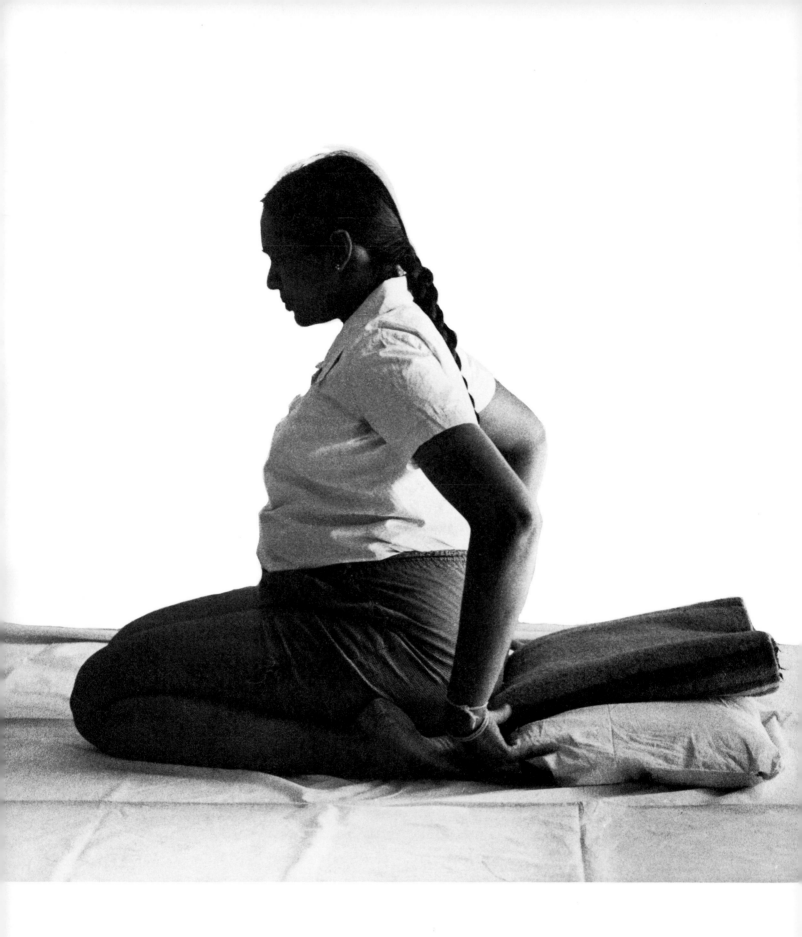

supta vīrāsana

Kneel down, sit on your heels.

By the way, do you remember how painful this simple sitting was when you started practicing?

And feel how pleasant and relaxing it is now.

May this always encourage you.

Now, keeping your feet extended, open your knees and sit between your open legs.

In the beginning, it may be a little difficult to bring your buttocks to rest on the ground.

Pull toward you folded blankets or a pillow you've kept near at hand and . . .

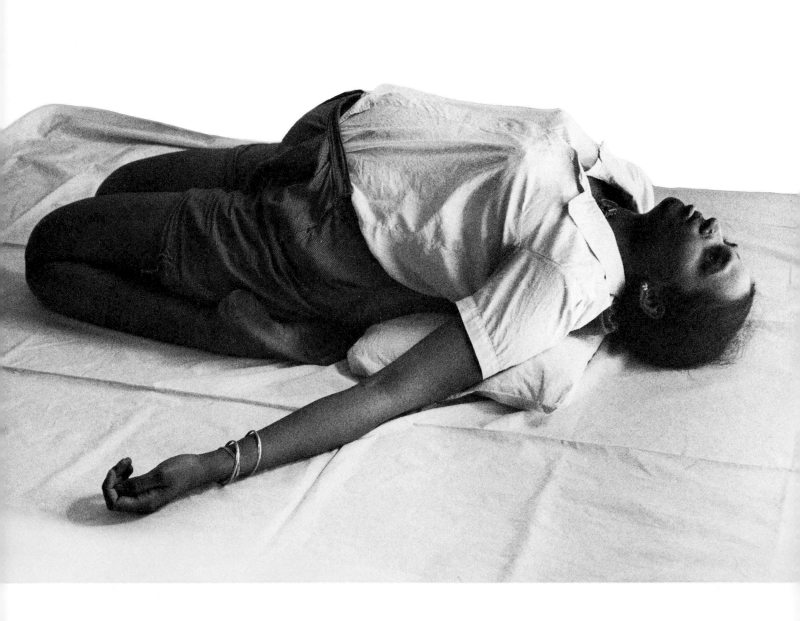

Resting your body first on your hands, then on your elbows,
lower your back very slowly
and bring it to rest on the blankets.

Blankets or pillows are essential.
Only then will your chest open, your pelvis relax, and
deep, spontaneous breathing begin.

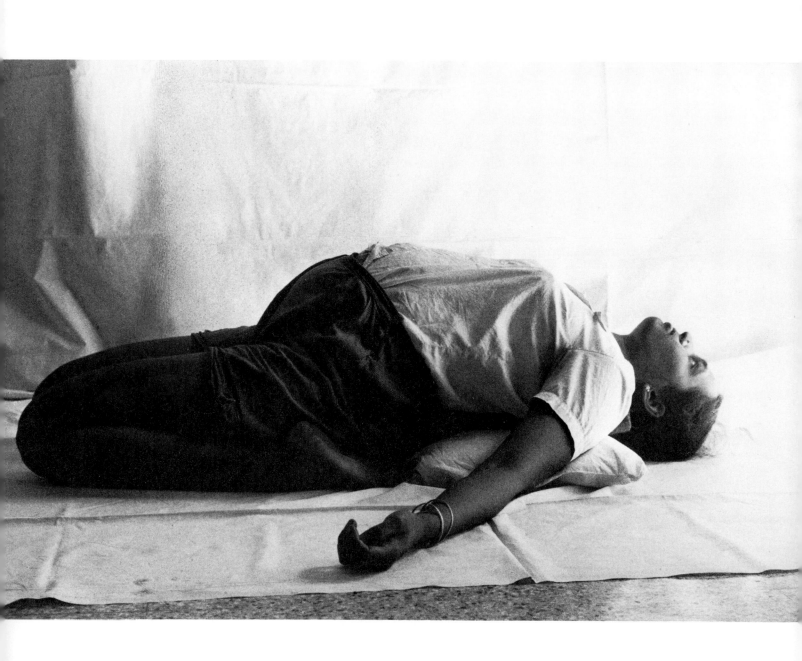

In the beginning, there may be pain.

Pain? No. Tension, and then, of course, resistance in the thighs.

But now you know what to make of it, how to cope with it. Open, and wait until deep breathing starts by *itself*.

Yes, nothing to do.
Just be there and open.
Feel how your chest is free,
and your hands,
and your neck.

One point: keep *lower jaw* and *tongue* free and relaxed.

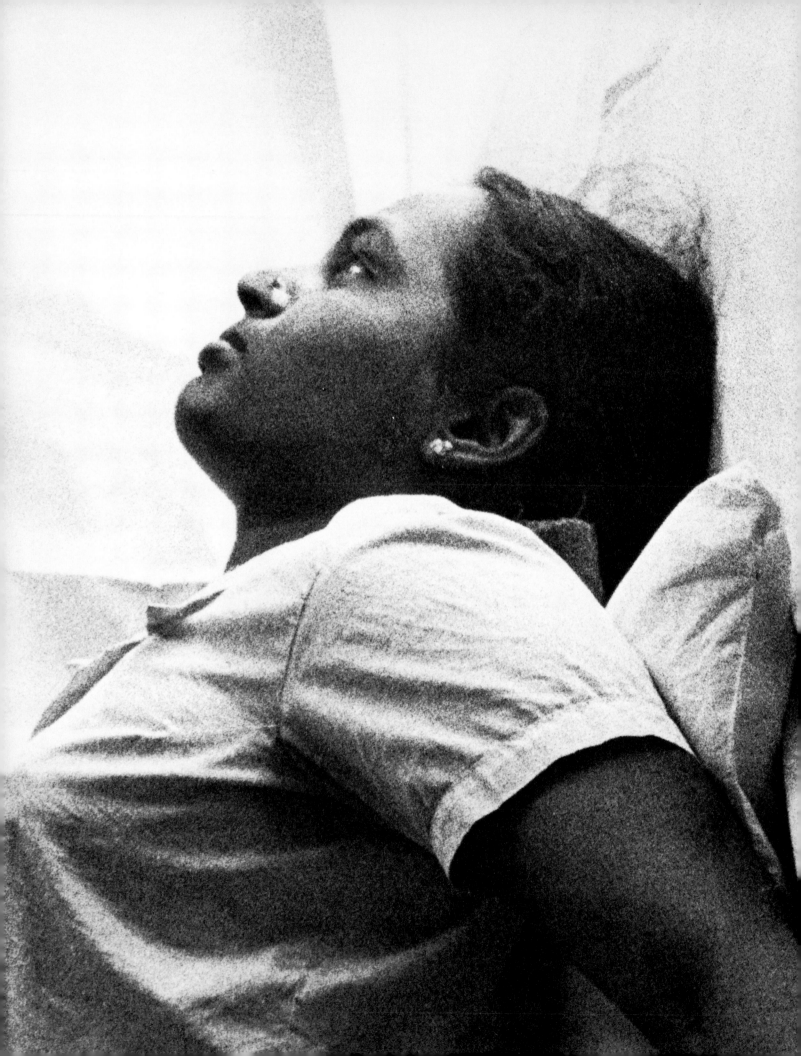

Nothing to do.
Just be.

Enjoy, enjoy the peace.

And yet, soon, one step further,
greater, yes, deeper peace
there is to be.

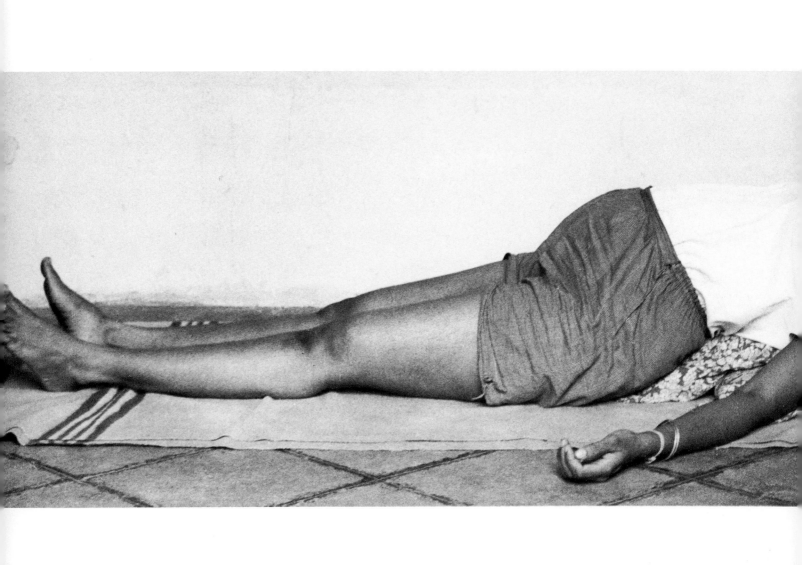

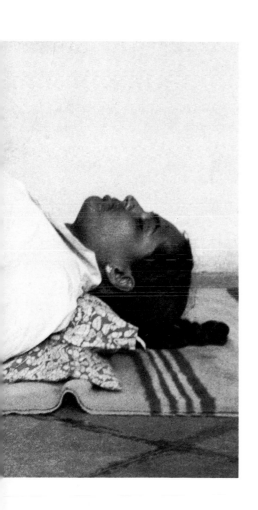

śavāsana

Śavāsana, indeed,
is the conclusion.
And Śavāsana means . . .
the corpse!

Death, a culmination!
Of course, it is the necessary conclusion
but . . .
does it mean that
I am going to die?

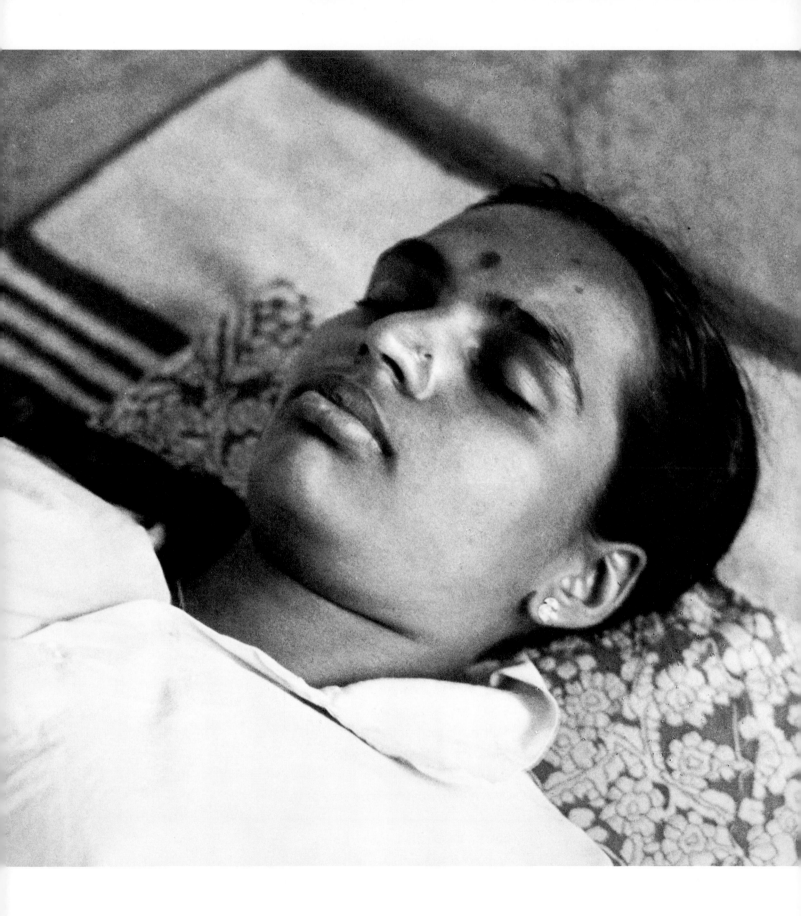

Of course, you will die.
Someday.
When you are very old.
But that is not now.

Who is going to die today?

Wait . . .
Your feet disentangled
and your legs stretched out,
pillow nicely arranged so that your head
comes to rest upon it
with no more tensions in your neck,
none in your throat,
with lower jaw *and tongue* fully relaxed
and hands open and free . . .

Listen inside.
Look within . . .

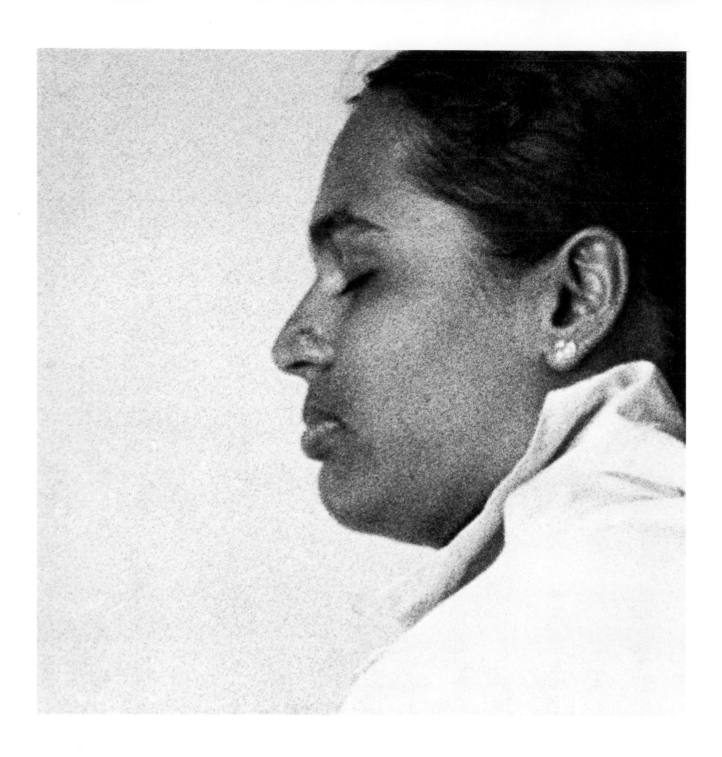

170

Where is this *I*, where is this *me*,
where is this elusive person?
Gone.
Tensions?
Yes, tensions, nothing more.
Such pains and fears
and sorrows
for nothing!
No thing. Or, rather, no.
Breathing,
sweet breathing.
And with its ebb and flow
no longer separate or lost
or alone, but floating,
dancing,
one with all.

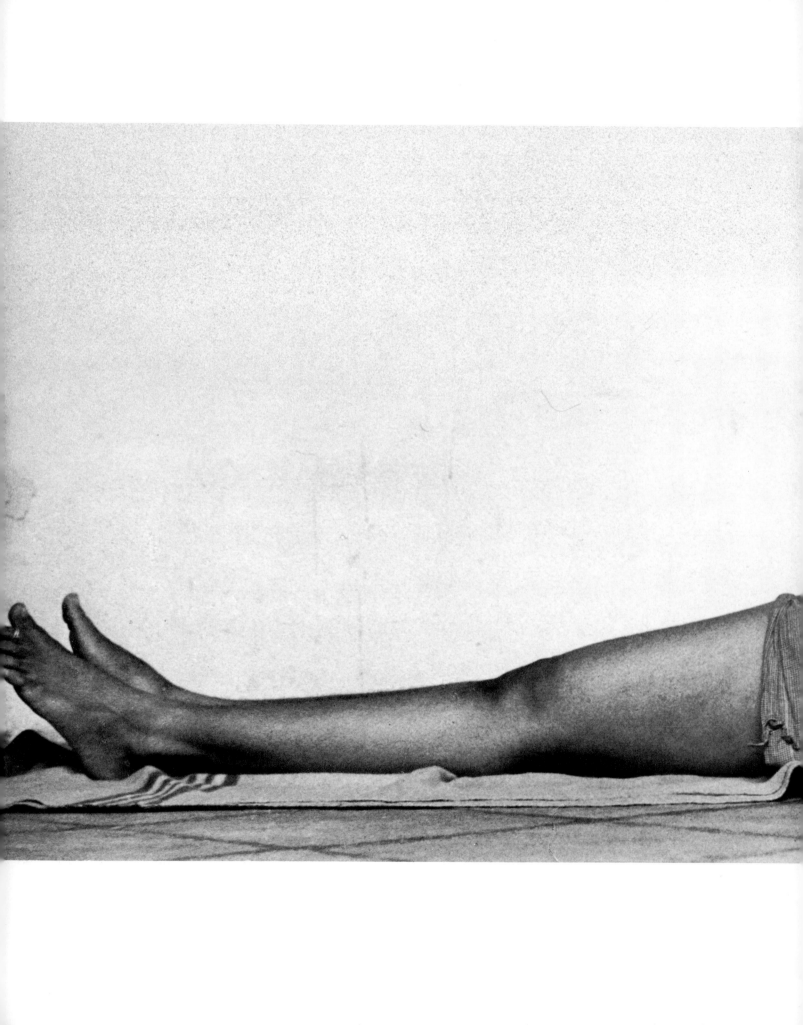

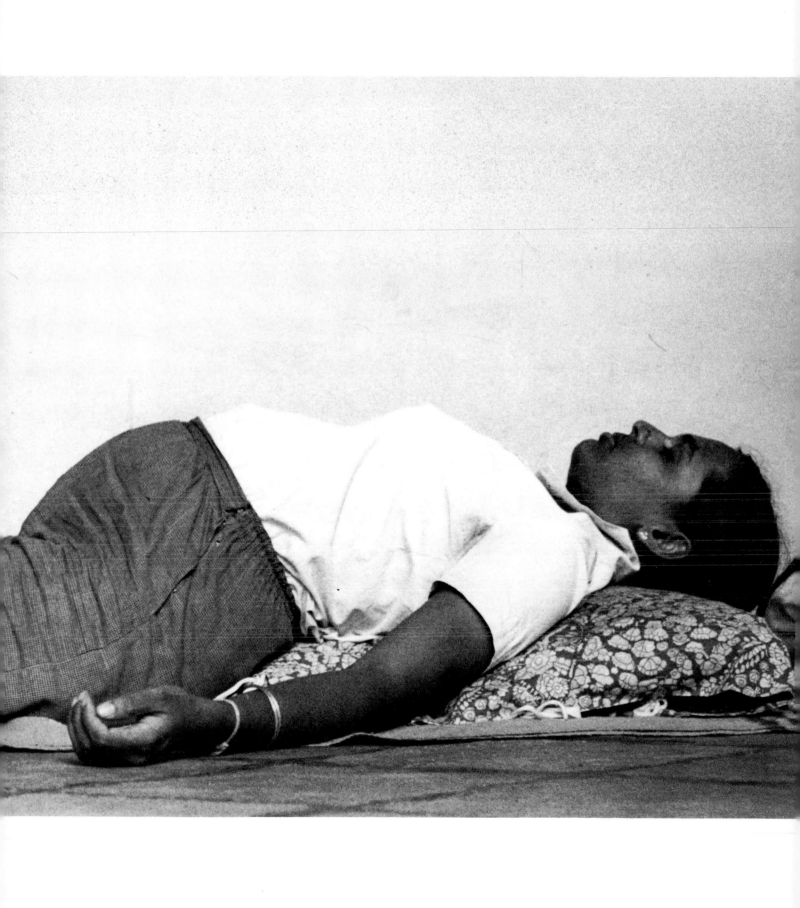

hints

—Right or wrong?
—No, no! Right or left.
  Or, rather, right and left.
  Each one in time.
  In tune.

                              —Sukhananda

At this point, you expect, usually, general principles, rules.

But Yoga is practice. It is personal experience.

It is truth. But a kind of truth you can hardly expect to find in books.

And then, Yoga is a way of freedom. Therefore, rules . . .

—Yoga, a way of freedom? Is it not, rather, a way of discipline?

It *is* a way of discipline. Freedom *through* discipline. But a discipline that comes from within. Not one that has been forced upon you from outside.

Within, outside . . .

There we are, trapped again.

This is what happens when one speaks.

Indeed, one who knows does not talk.

And, therefore, rules, principles?

They were there all along.

How could principles live apart from action?

Everything is one. There is no two.

One! Like water and salt in the deep sea,

like lovers lost in love.

One! As breathing is one with Āsanas.

Body *and* mind. Are they two?

Stop thinking. Stop asking.

Practice. Practice.

Never expect to reach truth through questions.

Is not the taste of wine in drinking?

The mere reading of a menu,

will it ever feed you?

1

Go slowly. Don't try to jump.
Patience is the greatest of all virtues.
And then, is it not Time you are trying to understand?
Faster, faster!
Is it not the music of the day?
While a Master always says
slowly, slowly.

2

Perfect action is complete,
carried out from beginning to end without a break.
And, indeed, beginning and end . . .

3

In a child, in a yogi,
in a baby,
everything moves and breathes together.
The pointing of a finger
actually originates in the opposite foot.
While most of you
is nothing but bits and pieces.

4

Strength . . . You know, now, that, ultimately,
it never conquers anything.
How vulgar, how coarse, compared to intelligence.

5

Breathing . . .
All important. And yet not *yours*.
Inhaling, exhaling. Taking and giving.
To give is yours.
Taking is not.

Be happy to receive. Knowing that what you get is never what you expected.

Therefore, give, give! Exhale, exhale!

And see how, the moment you are totally empty

something takes place

that makes you full.

Spontaneously. Effortlessly.

6

Same postures every day. And in the same order.

But that must be boring!

The same, yes. And always new.

For ever and ever. Indefinitely.

7

As time goes by and we grow old

our movements become rigid and restricted,

our actions narrow and petty.

This is the voice of age. The way to death.

Mechanical, blind repetition can only dull.

But when there is profound attention

one never stops seeing deeper and deeper.

And intelligence sharpens more and more.

8

In any posture you can cheat.

In Paschimottānāsana, for instance, you can bend your knees.

Not much, of course. No one would know.

You see what I mean: the tiny dishonesty you get away with every day.

Well, cheat if you like. Impress your friends.

They might think you've made it.

But your teacher knows. For there is no detail he could possibly miss.

He may reprimand you. Or he may wait.
Until you understand that, ultimately, you can cheat no one
but yourself.

9

Imitating . . .
We, really, do nothing else.
The child imitates his parents.
Parents, themselves, used to imitate their parents.
Who, unfortunately, could not even walk or stand properly.
This is why we all need a master at some point:
someone who stands and walks
the right way.

But beware:
a Master! Then one feels great!
And to follow, of course, is so pleasant.
To imitate and to understand. There is quite a difference.
Monkeys and sheep, on one side.
And Man, on the other.
Yes, make sure you understand
the *way* your master indicates.
Lest you soon merely eat the same food and
dress like him.

10

Your *mind* . . .
Ah, the strange, the terrible animal!
Unless you, constantly, keep an eye on this ape, you miss
your time.

When you meet with some serious difficulty with an Āsana,
have you noticed the *voice inside?*
How it grumbles? Not to say more.

When your teacher corrects your posture,
do you feel hurt? Do you start to argue?
Do you swear you'll revenge?
Or that, one day, he will fall for you?

Do you feel elated when your posture is praised
and utterly depressed when criticized
or merely ignored?
In other words, are you truly enjoying your practicing
or still feeding your ego?

Oh, yes, see, see
all that is, constantly, going on in your mind.

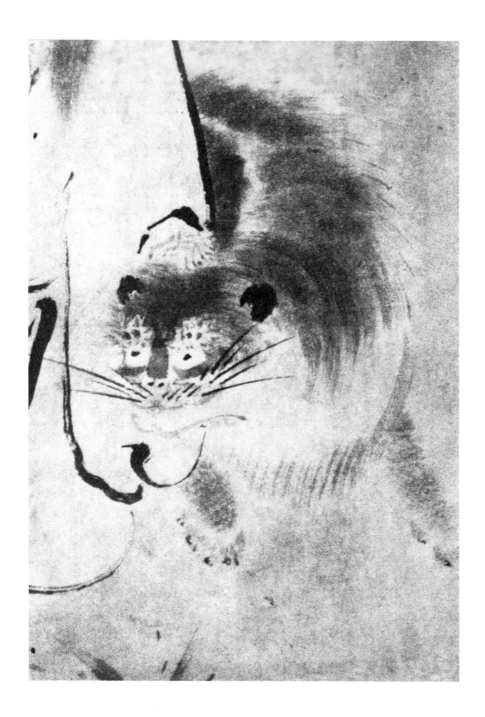

Altogether it is a difficult
even a dangerous affair.
The animal we are after is really ferocious.
Such teeth! Such claws!
It takes all the skill of a true hunter,
all his patience, his caution,
his knowledge and his love
to help you tame that tiger.

Ah, yes, beware. For, once wounded,
the animal becomes even more terrible.
Who knows what it will do.

And, no killing, of course.
Tiger skins, no, no.
That is not it at all.
We want the animal alive.
Bouncing, happy, friendly.

Yes, it takes a perfect man.
Therefore, choose your teacher carefully.
If he tries to impress you with his postures
make sure that he does not need your admiration to feel great.
Indeed, he ought to be concerned
with *your* difficulties,
not with *his* own achievements.
Definitely a sportsman will not do.
What if you keep expanding your chest, year after year,
and still remain speechless or even blush
in front of a policeman or anyone with a big voice?
What if you can stand on your head
and still begin to cry, at night, in the forest?

Yes, be careful, be careful.
One may become a great acrobat
and still remain
a little child.

Ultimately, Chuang Tsü once again comes to mind.

Indeed, wisdom knows no borders.

Here is a little story he tells and which, I am sure, will make the point clear.

One day, Lie Y. was demonstrating his skill in archery for Pai-huen Wu-jen.

Lie Y. would draw his mighty bow at full arm's length with such skill that not one drop would overflow, the moment he let the arrow go, from a cup full of water which he had placed on his elbow.

And so swift and fast was he that no sooner had the first arrow gone, than a second and then a third would already be flying away.

And, all the while, he would remain motionless as a stone statue.

—Not bad. Not bad at all, said Pai-huen. Well done indeed. But this is still "doing."

—What do you mean, still "doing"? exclaimed Lie Y.

—You see, said Pai-huen, your shooting is excellent, no doubt. But this is not yet pure shooting.

—Pure shooting . . . ?

—It is still your shooting. Tomorrow, come with me. I know a little place, in the hills, where you may possibly attain pure shooting.

And so the next day, before dawn, they climbed up a very high mountain, until they reached a small rocky terrace, overlooking a terrible precipice, at least three thousand feet deep.

Turning his back to the void, Pai-huen started walking backward.

And only when he felt his heels were in the void did he stop! Bowing to Lie Y.:

—Come and join me, said he very quietly.

Poor Lie Y. He had fallen to the ground.

A cold sweat was running all over his body, down to his very heels.

Then said Pai-huen:

— The Perfect Man, my friend,
if he soars to the top of heaven
or sinks to the bottom of the abyss,
if he reaches to the eight poles
of the great universe,
neither his mind not his breathing
is affected in the least.
And there you are, sweating, shaking with fear,
and about to faint for so little?
The freedom, the command over yourself that
you felt you had achieved
must be very superficial, I am afraid.

Can you take classes in laughing?
Someone says something funny
and you laugh.
Where did it hit?
Your ear? Your mind?
And what is it that laughed?
Your chest? Your ribs? Your diaphragm?

—Yes. Yes, I suppose I begin to see.

—Oh really!

—But, these Asanas, am I to perform all of them every day? I shall never have time . . .

—Time? Yes, time, indeed. Be happy: no, you won't have to perform them all. At least not every day. Shall we say two or three? Will that do? But then, do them every day.

Two or three every day.

Then I would not be surprised if three, soon, become four. Four become five . . .

One day you will do them all. And ask for more!

A journey of ten thousand miles . . .

Now, on the contrary, it may happen that you begin with great zest and enthusiasm.

You do the whole series twice a day.

But soon, you miss a few postures.

And then you miss more and more.

Until you give up the whole thing altogether.

You see, enthusiasm is fine. But, like boiling water, it must end up being cold. Or even freeze.

All right. It does not matter.

If once you tried, one day or another you will try again.

A little wiser

hopefully.

—So, I do not have to do them all? Good. I feel better. But then, tell me, which Āsanas are good for me?

—Good for you?

—You see, my feet get cold easily in winter. And, after a heavy meal, my stomach . . .

—My friend, my friend . . . Yoga is neither good for this nor for that. Some books, indeed, even some teachers recommend this posture in case of poor sleep, that one if you have trouble with your motions,

and that posture, they say, unfailingly prevents graying of the hair, relieves hiccups, purifies the breath, and, ultimately, cools the brain.

What a poor understanding of Yoga!

Analyzing, specializing,

running after goals . . .

Yoga teaches you detachment and oneness.

It tries to make you see that in the part is the whole.

In each Āsana,

indeed, is the whole of Yoga.

Tell me: the air you breathe,
that fills your chest,
is it meant for your heart?
Or is it not rather best for your head?
Will it do good to your liver?
To your right eye or your little finger?

—Well, I am afraid I don't see the point. And I feel that you are very rude not to answer my questions. But, then, what is the best time?

—The best time?

—Is it better to practice in the morning or in the evening?

—Morning *and* evening.

—What! Twice a day!

—All right. Morning, I would say, would be fine.

—Oh, really? I had thought evening would be better.

Questions, questions.
Why don't you start!
Two or three. At any time.
But do them every day.

The rest will follow.
And, as I said already, a time will come when you do them all
and ask for more.

More?
No doubt, you are on the way.
But more and more, is that not still the voice of the child? The
craving, the cupidity?
More and more, where will it end?

Therefore, at one point, less and less.
Deeper and deeper.
No doubt now you make progress.

Someday, possibly, one only.
But so beautifully, so slowly.

And then, a day will come when Yoga is no longer something
you do twice a day.
It is there all the time.
Indeed, it was there always.
Whatever you do is Āsanas to you.
The way you walk
or sit or stand or take a cup,
the way you wave your hand or turn your eyes,
it all tells . . .

Ease and grace,
freedom and harmony.
Not strength but forcefulness.
Complete openness.

You are not far
from oneness.

Which Āsanas are good for me? How many . . . ?

A time will come when questions stop.
And then, surprisingly,
often in a strange way,
answers come.

Isn't the way
full of mystery?

the secret

The sun
does not shine purposely.
It expects neither praise nor rewards.
It shines.
That's all.
Rather, it burns.
And it is the very excess
of its all-consuming joy
which keeps overflowing
constantly.

— Sukhananda

1.

— Yes. Yes, indeed. But then you see I am pregnant. I want to know!

— You want to know, *what?*

— What I am to do when it comes?

— What *I* am to do when *it* comes. Beautiful! Beautiful! See how truth will out! This charming, innocent mouth has just voiced it. And you *think* that you don't know? *I* and *it*. What am *I* to do when *it* comes. It is all there, in those few words.

— . . . ?

— Something will be there, will happen. Something will take place. Be with *it*. That is all. Be *it*. No separation, no refusal. Do not try to run away, to stop, to deny. And, mostly, no fear! *It* is there. Let *it* take *its* own course. Let *it* take care of *itself*. Rather, allow *it* to take you there.

2

—Now, really, you are not kind! You are a wicked man. You never answer my questions. I was quite prepared to do Yoga . . .

—Do. Do. Practice. Practice.

—And you only confuse me. You must tell me!

—I must tell you *what*? Which Āsana you are to do in case contractions come too often? At which point you are to start standing on your head? Which posture is likely to relieve back pain? This is what you want to know?

—But yes, of course!

—I'm terribly sorry, my dear child, but this is not at all the way it works.

—But, then, how does it work?

—I don't know.

—What do you mean, you don't know!

—Honestly, I don't know. But that it works, oh yes, this I know.

3

—Accept that it will be a surprise. A wonderful surprise. Something totally different from anything you could ever think of.

Yes, when it comes, let it happen.

Everything will be all right.

All troubles come from the mind, from having ideas, from trying to imagine.

Yes, stop thinking.

And, mostly, stop expecting.

Expectation always is a lie which can meet only with frustration.

4

—What do you mean, stop expecting! But I *am* expecting!

—Oh yes, of course. I'm terribly sorry. Certainly I never meant
. . . Then let me tell you a secret. A great, a deep, a wonderful
secret.

—A secret? At last!

—You see . . .

Love, o love,
you must have gone mad
that, so furiously, you get at me.
But yes, hit me, do destroy
this terrified, petty little me
so that nothing's left
but Thee.

— St. Izine de Treves

— You see, ultimately, the truth is that you are afraid.

— Well . . . yes. I am a little scared.

— A little? You are terrified.

Why . . . I am very much afraid.

— All right. But why? .

— People say it is so painful.

— People say . . . What is that to you! The fact is that the way *people* look at childbirth, nowadays, in your countries is rather strange. It has become a medical affair. And, in the most privileged of these advanced countries, a matter of surgery! But then, tell me, is it an illness, a malady?

— But . . . of course not.

— Isn't it a most natural, normal affair? As natural and simple as taking food or walking or sleeping?

— Well . . . yes. Of course. But then, there is risk.

— Ah, risk. Yes. There is risk. But risk is everywhere. Risk *is* life. Deny risk, try to protect yourself against it, and you cut yourself off from life. Accept it and you are free. The moment you accept it, nothing will ever touch you! Start to protect yourself and you will be hurt again and again. But although there *is* risk (far less, actually, than people try to make you believe), it is not risk you are afraid of.

—What am I afraid of, then?

—You are afraid. That is all. And you project this fear all around: the hospital might not be properly equipped. Or, the doctor might not be there in time.

—Yes.

—I shall try to make it clearer so that you, really, can see. Suppose you go to the cinema and see a thriller, a movie that very much frightens you. You are so moved, the fear becomes so strong that, at times, you stop looking. And, once you are home, in your bed, you can't sleep. Do you follow?

—Oh, yes, it happened to me recently. I got so scared that I could not sleep for three nights. I even had to keep a night light.

—Ah, you see.

—I lost my appetite and would not even go to the basement where it is so dark.

—There you are! Terrible fear, indeed. But then, as you may know, there is another kind of fear.

—Another?

—When you were looking at the movie, the cinema, I mean the *building* might have caught fire. Were you afraid of that?

—I never even thought of it.

—Indeed. Then, you can see these two kinds of fear. The fear originated by the movie and the fear of fire. The first one, shall we say, is purely imaginary. While the fear of fire is real. Since fire, in a cinema, although very rare, is a true possibility.

—Oh, I suppose I begin to see.

—Isn't it extraordinary that the imaginary, illusory fear, the fear created by the movie, should be far more real to you than the so-called real fear, the fear of the fire?

—Indeed. That's absurd.

—Absurd, but there it is. And this is exactly what happens in childbirth. You are afraid, as you were telling me, but not at all of real dangers. You are not at all concerned with possible real difficulties such as infection or hemorrhage. Actually, the fear that catches hold of you is the same fear that stops children from going into darkness which is, to them, full of tigers and crocodiles. It is the same fear, again, that makes women faint at the mere sight of a tiny little spider or a harmless mouse. Fear is in your mind. On the screen. It is the fear of the movie, not the fear of any real fire.

—I see. Oh, yes, now I begin to understand.

—Tell me: the first time a young man kissed you, you were afraid? Try to remember.

—Well . . . Yes, you are right. I was afraid.

—Was it painful?

—Oh, no!

—The suffering was so great, it hurt so much that, never again, you swore . . .

—Now you are laughing at me.

—Again, try to remember: the first night you surrendered to your lover, you were afraid, were you not?

—I was trembling all over. How my heart was beating!

—And the pain was beyond words?

—Oh, dear me, no!

—But, try to see. Was pleasure there, right from the start?

—. . . no.

—Did not pleasure, actually, start the moment fear was over and you began to let go, surrender?

—Yes. Yes. Oh, again, I see. But then, do you mean to say . . .

—Yes . . . ?

—That giving birth and making love . . .

—Yes . . . ?

—Are one and the same experience?

—There you are! Yes, indeed.

—Oh!

—Did I not promise you a secret? A wonderful secret?

—Childbirth . . . a sexual experience . . .

—The culmination of sex. Rather, the culmination of love. Since sex alone, deprived of its emotional component, is purely animal and thus, frustrating. Lust. Appetite. Purely physical. Dry and empty. And petty. But, yes, childbirth is the culmination of love. Emotionally and sexually.

—I can't believe it. And yet it seems so obvious.

—Are not the same organs, the same parts of the body involved?

—Yes, of course.

—And, you know that when sex is forced on you against your will, your consent, it turns into pain?

—Yes.

—Similarly, try to fight, to refuse, to stop the whole loving process of childbirth, and you experience the unbearable, excruciating pain of being raped.

—I see. I see! Childbirth and making love . . .

—You never thought of it that way, did you?

—Never! Never.

—So, you see, it is fear. Nothing but fear. The fear of something much stronger than *you* which takes command. *You,* little *you* being carried away, overwhelmed, swept away. Or, rather, swept along. And *little you,* of course, is terrified. When did you experience that for the first time?

—In sex, in love, as you said.

—And before that?

— . . .

—In your own birth.

—Really!

—Yes. A fantastic power taking *hold* of you. The contractions of the womb! Which were madly pushing you toward life.

—But then, sex and birth . . .

—One and the same process. The power of sex, of love and their fascination is nothing but the nostalgia of this tremendous adventure. Altogether terrifying and tantalizing. And, since giving birth and being born are one and the same experience, you cannot but be both frightened and fascinated. You see, in a pregnant woman, the past is reactivated. She becomes, again, in many ways, a little girl. She wants support. She wants love. She is afraid.

Of the newness, the unknown. Just like the little child, the little baby she once was.

—I see.

—But once you keep in mind the first kiss, the first night with your lover, why should you be afraid?

—The same fear . . . And then, the same heart-breaking longing, the same expectation.

—Are not women, in this case, said to be *expecting?*

—Why, yes!

—And then, there is a proof that childbirth, indeed, is sex, is love.

—A proof?

—Breathing.

—Breathing, yes. Breathing, as you may know, is one. And many.

You laugh, you giggle. You cry, you scream. You shout in anger. You tenderly whisper. Or you yawn.

Breathing, breathing, breathing tuned to your many moods.

And then, of course, there is talking. Breathing becomes thoughts.

And then, there is singing, poetry.

Breathing. Again. Coming from deeper.

Is that all?

There is yet another.

Totally different. Coming from much farther,

a wind that comes from far, far away,

from sacred, distant wonderlands.

A wind? Rather a gentle breeze. That is, to men, even dearer, warmer than the warmth of the sun.

—A wind? A gentle breeze?

—The secret whisper of love: the moment the god touches you and you respond, your breathing tells the tale.

Its rhythm changes. And its music.

It all becomes so deep, so slow, so moving.

It is something no sensitive ear, indeed, could miss.

If, on the contrary, you won't respond, your breathing, again, betrays you: here is something you can neither fake nor imitate. You cannot pretend.

It does not depend on your will. It is not yours.

The moment Eros is there, he takes command.
Takes hold of you.

Oh, this caress, this whisper . . .
So light when it is born, when it begins,
so sweet, so deep, so slow.
Heavy, weary with tenderness
and weak and shy and shivering.
Love . . .
But soon it grows
into a wild, all-powerful wind that tolerates no barriers.
A wind? A storm! Raging, rushing.
At times, crying, moaning.
A song of want, of dear longing.
Utter despair or ecstasy?
At times no one could say.

And this very breathing, this panting
which is the voice of love,
which is the song of Man
is there, in women, the moment labor starts.
The same rhythm, the same music, the same raving madness,
the very same awesome beauty.
No sensitive ear could miss it.

A great god is there
who holds you in his sway.
You are frightened, panic-stricken?
Of course. Such a lover, such a passion, such a fire.

Can you fight gods? Can you say no?
And why should you, now that you know?

—Yes. Yes, now I think I understand . . . the fear and . . . every-thing.

—You do? I am glad. And then, in case you still might think it is all the creation of a mad mind, of a poet, do listen to what a *woman* has to say.

Do listen carefully, since each word is full of significance.
And since she expresses herself so beautifully:

the sun is within me and so is the moon
—Kabir

The celebration of birth begins with a sudden yet gentle release of the primordial waters. My body is awakened to a new movement within, not yet rhythmic, but strong enough to begin the breathing and the inner meditation that my teacher has given me. I continue to breathe while bathing and wrapping myself in a towel, when suddenly I am seized by an incredible tremor arising from the depths of my body. I hold to the window's ledge and, while watching the familiar mango tree in the yard become unfamiliar, my entire being is convulsed and drawn into itself.

I sense immediately that I will be continuously absorbed by this passionate movement until it culminates itself. I am now totally taken by this energy that is not separate from myself. With each rise of its force I feel the passage that I have become opening itself ever more and more, each breath seems to uncover a new space. There is only expansion now and no limitation is endured. The event tolerates no measuring, will not be in any way contained. It seems on the contrary to have contained my whole self. There is no choice to be had, the meditation is the dance.

A natural birth is a manifestation of spontaneous expression and cannot be schooled, urged, or thrust upon a mode of living that is not natural. It requires only a clear channel, a body in health, a mind in understanding, a whole being that is totally open. When the intelligence of the body is awakened, as through the practice of yoga, it will guide the woman throughout the pregnancy, making her feel perhaps more in touch with her self than ever before. She is then close to her own nature and ready to flow with the movement of birth when it begins.

The breath will move evenly throughout each phase. Conscious maintenance of the breath can be the means through which the woman retains the pulse of what is happening. She is then one with all that waxes and wanes, rises and falls, inhales and exhales. All of creation is with her as she becomes the very passage for life itself. And when the moment arrives to receive the fruit of her love, she is truly there in that silent, joyous space to meet the small one with reverence and wonder.

Birth can be seen now, not as a procedure separate from the living of each day, but rather as a proceeding from the very roots of it. The greatest preparation that can be made for the birth of a child is to allow for the constant arising of birth in one's self. And this arising can take place only in a space that is clear and free of expectation.

The sublime energy that, when trusted to pass freely, will move the womb to open and empty itself, bringing forth the new life, will also sweep through the being of the mother, giving rise to birth and rebirth simultaneously and at each instant. The intensity of childbirth brings the supreme moment in which the usual hold on one's self can be shaken and undone. One falls into the exultation of life as it lives itself. Birth then is the occasion of vibrating with the universal rhythm, a moment to feel the perfect accord of what is below with what is above, a merging with the cosmic dance.

Who wrote these lines?

A mystic? A saint? A great poet living in some distant country, centuries ago?

A great poet, certainly.

But one of you: Maria Rosenstone, a young American who lives near San Francisco.

Indeed, she spent two full years in India, became a vegetarian, and devoted herself to the practice of Yoga.

Did she become a recluse?

No!

She became a mother. Had two children

and talks and writes from personal experience, the reason you may trust every word she says.

Therefore, when the time comes
when the sweet torment of labor begins
don't be afraid.
— I hope it will help you when the time comes.
— Indeed, it will.
— When the sweet torment, labor, starts you won't be afraid?
— No, no.
— You will keep in mind these words of Maria? You will remember the first kiss?
— Yes, yes.
— And, all along, you will keep thinking, feeling
it's love
nothing but love
and this mad lover
fighting his way
through me.

love bless you

At times, it may have been confusing:
feet, hands, arms, legs, eyes,
mind, body
and breathing!
How am I ever to make it all work together!
I?
Who am I? My legs? My eyes? My mind? My . . .
Yes. Who am I?
Not a bad question, by the way.
Did not Socrates already say:
"Know yourself."
Or, rather:
"Know your Self."

Yes, yes, who am I?
Breathing?
Possibly.
Let me tell you: it is a great mystery.

—Breathing, a mystery? But breathing is taking oxygen, says the biologist. Where do you see any mystery?

—Oxygen, yes, says the physician. But don't forget the lungs.

Oxygen, lungs.
Is that all?
Let me tell you one last little story.

One day, a man who was deaf saw someone playing the piano.

—What is this fool doing! said the man who could not hear, greatly surprised.

And, after very hard *thinking:*

—The poor fellow must have trouble with his fingers. Rheumatism. Or arthritis. He must be doing exercises prescribed by his therapist.

Yes, you see, lungs, oxygen, most probably something must be missing. What?

Love?

Ah, possibly.

Are we not told that love is everywhere?

And then, now you may understand that taking classes, doing breathing exercises, well . . .

When you are in your lover's arms, does it ever occur to you that you ought to do deep breathing?

When the sweet madness of love carries you away, do you ever stop and think

. . . now the little book was telling me . . . at this stage use breathing technique number three . . . No! Wait . . . number . . . No! No . . . four . . . six? Not yet! Oh, wait, wait, oh . . . yes, oh yes! Oh yes!

But then, love is shy.
It wants intimacy, half-lights, twilight
and quietness and silence.
Therefore, love
in hospitals
under the glaring lights
with all sorts of people watching you,
a drip in one arm, a needle in your back . . .
Difficult.
Very, very difficult indeed.

Then it turns into its very opposite:
rape
and its excruciating pain.
Plus the utter humiliation
of public defecation.

Ah, yes, remember, remember
love, nothing but love.
And its folly.
And this mad lover
within me.

Within?
Inside?
Of course: where is the storm
but in my chest!
What is this furious wind
but my own breath!

down to earth!

Before we part for good, a few very practical points.

lying in bed, during labor?

Is it all right to be in bed during labor?

Well, you are not sick, are you? And childbirth is not a disease.

Therefore, far better to stand, walk, sit, kneel.

And, at times, of course, lie down.

In fact, do whatever you feel like.

Trust your body. Allow it to play. And do whatever it feels like.

For, indeed, don't forget: it's love! It's love!

A bed? Why not the floor?

Beds are far too narrow, restricted.

In order to stretch out, to play, your body wants far more space than any bed can provide.

Kneeling.

Now that your ankles are free and you can enjoy the deeply relaxing effect of kneeling, do.

With knees wide open to accommodate your big stomach.

In front of you, a pile of cushions.

And lean on them with arms wide open.

Lie on your back?

Yes. But never for too long. Since it is so uncomfortable for your child.

Never *flat on your back* anyway. Rather use a pillow as you have been instructed after Śīrṣāsana and in Supta Vīrāsana.

Lie on your side?

Yes, far better.

Rather, this is the perfect way of lying

during labor

and all through the last weeks of pregnancy.

But the technique is very precise.

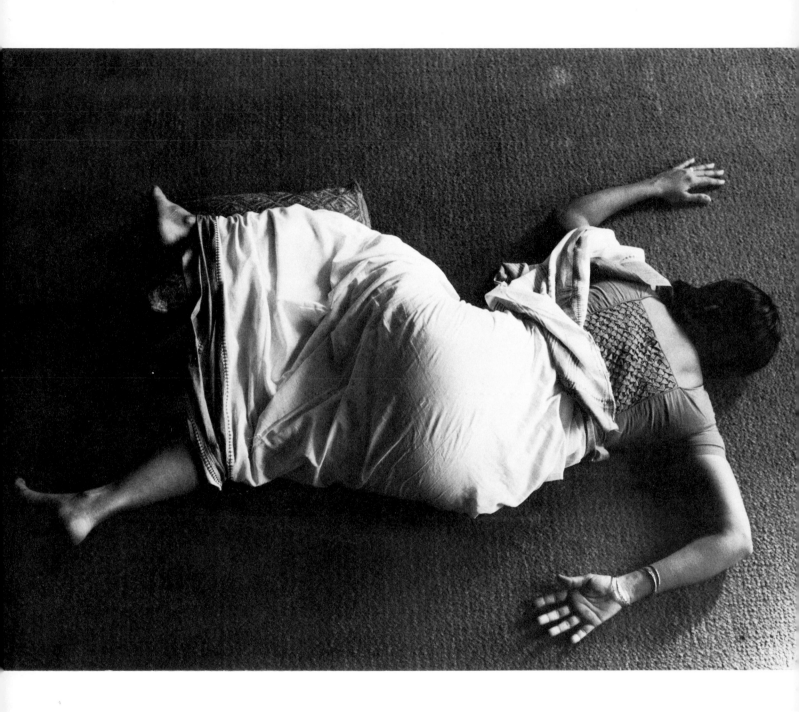

Take a good look at the pictures and notice:

Arms: perpendicular to the axis of your body.

Forearms: again perpendicular to your arms.

Hands: when lying on your *right* side, as shown in the photograph, your right hand is *behind,* palm facing the sky.

Your left hand, on the contrary, is *in front of you, palm down,* touching, caressing, as it were, the ground with *great sensitivity.*

Legs: your *left* knee is *up,* close to your *left elbow.* Thigh at right angle to the body. Calf at right angle to the thigh.

When you get very near to the end of labor, put one or two pillows under this *left* knee in order to better support it. It will open your pelvis effortlessly.

Axis: the transversal axis of your pelvis, from hip to hip is *perpendicular* to the ground and to the axis of your *shoulders*, which are parallel to the ground.

With each *exhale,* let go, surrendering to the earth, your mother, heaving a deep sigh of love and well-being.

This emptying of your chest and your self brings your *left* shoulder closer and closer to the ground, accentuating the *twist* in your spine.

Which brings on quite naturally, *passively,* spontaneous, deeply relaxing *abdominal* breathing.

Of course, after lying on one side, turn over to the other.

You may notice also that, in this posture, your body looks very much like a *swastika,* the symbol of circulating life energy.

So many words for such a simple thing . . .

Indeed, the mind is so clumsy!

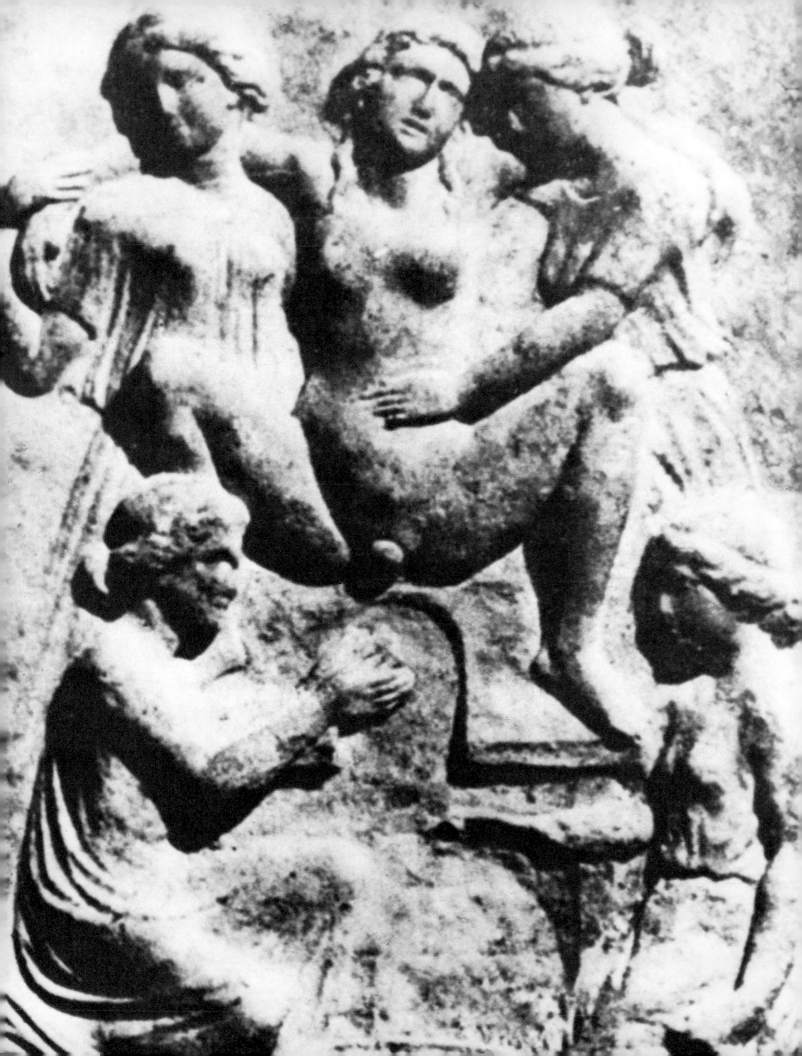

baby is about to be born

When the head of the baby begins to press hard on the perineum, what are you to do? Rather, what posture are you to take?

Let me point out what *not to do.*

For one thing, since you fully understand the importance of *feet* and *grounding,* stirrups that keep feet dangling in the air are to be discarded once and for all.

And then, at this stage, you are never to be *lying on your back.*

No one could pass stool or even water in this position. Far less can one help the baby being born.

Then, what are you to do?

Take any position that keeps your body *close to the vertical.*

You may recline against a wall. And far better against cushions and pillows.

Or you may be supported by friends or your husband, as you can see in the picture.

This Roman lady, on her very low wooden delivery bed, gets full support from her two friends.

Having her arms round their shoulders keeps her chest fully open, allowing free abdominal, diaphragmatic breathing.

You may notice also the very convenient aperture in the bed which is so useful for watching the perineum and catching the baby when it comes.

But even better than being supported by friends' shoulders, let the midwife or your *husband* sit *behind* you with legs wide open, offering to your *back* the support of her or his *chest.*

Here *both breathings harmonize.*

Thus this is the only way for your husband (or anyone) truly to participate and help you,

since, through *breathing in tune with you* he can give you his own energy.

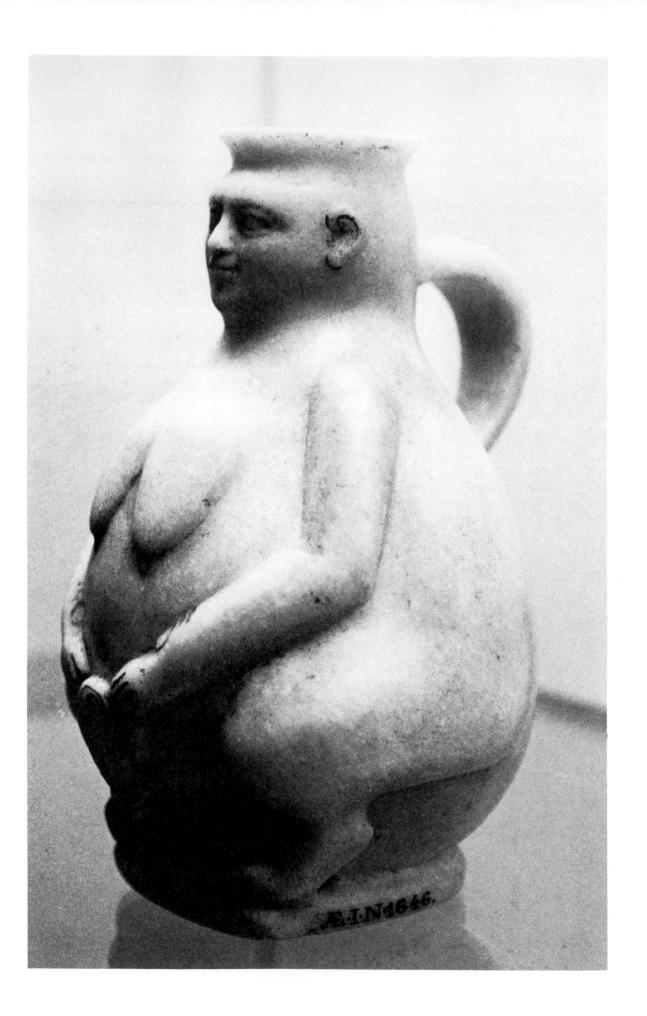

close to the vertical

What helps the baby to get through is *not the weight,*

but, indeed, this *all-powerful something* which makes trees, flowers, and plants grow *skyward.*

In India it is called *prana.*

The Chinese call it *chi.*

Although closely connected with breathing, it is neither air nor oxygen.

The Egyptians knew it also as is shown beautifully in this goddess of fertility.

She reminds us, for one thing, that man is half angel, half devil, half animal and half what someday might be called Man. For, indeed, her hind legs look very much like a dog's.

The enormous, round belly stands both for abdominal breathing and pregnancy.

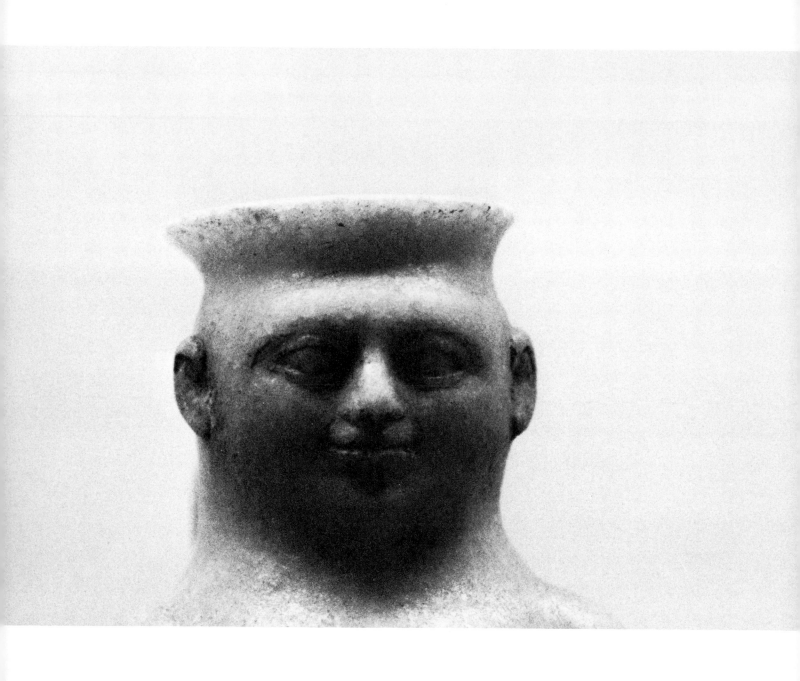

pulling or pushing?

Usually women are instructed to *pull* on their folded knees and to *push*.

Beautiful contradiction: either you *push* or you *pull*.

And the baby gets stuck, of course.

Pulling then, or pushing?

Pushing, of course, since only pushing opens your *back*,

which opens your chest and gives full, open play to your diaphragm and, at the same time, opens and relaxes your pelvic muscles and vulva.

In fact, if all goes well and you are really, totally free from *fears* and *tensions*, you are neither to pull nor push.

There is *nothing to do.* Just as in lovemaking.

Open and let go.

Surrender. Allow it to happen.

Being, merely, a witness.

A bewildered, raptured witness.

To your utter amazement you watch yourself and the baby being carried, as it were, by an uninterrupted, continuous, flowing, beautifully rhythmic process.

Yes: *nothing to do.*

Just be. And flow with the process.

The inner power

and the baby

have done it all for you.

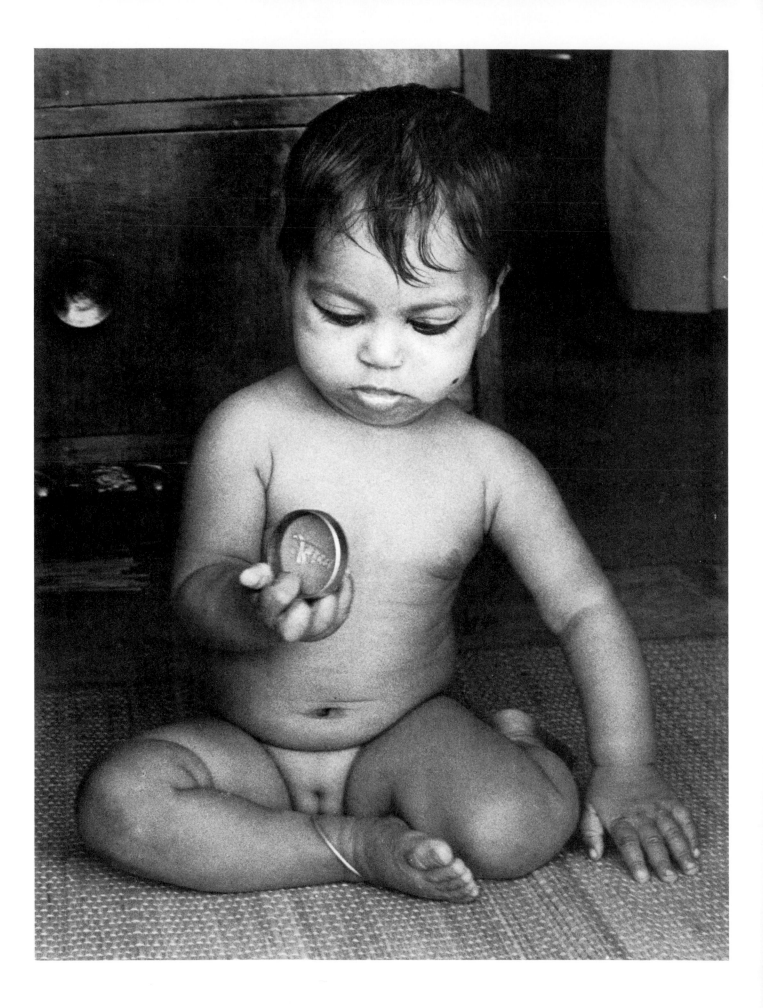

This one lesson you should never forget: the baby, not you, runs the show.

You must accept that there is far more to this newborn than you, generally, think.

It is not at all *that poor little thing* people take it to be.

Babies know.

Which means that, in education,

you are to learn,

not to teach.

In case you are not convinced and still feel so superior to children, take a good look at this lovely baby and try this very simple (!) Āsana in front of a mirror . . .

How are your shoulders?

Both on the same level and parallel to the ground?

Are *both* your buttocks touching the ground?

Or is not rather one of the two floating somewhere, up in the air?

Is the posture pleasant, comfortable, easy?

And how is your spine?

Does your trunk remind you of the noble pine tree, shooting straight to the sky?

Or is it a tormented, twisted, wind-battered bush that comes to mind?

Who's the master here?

You? Or the baby?

and who is vanita?

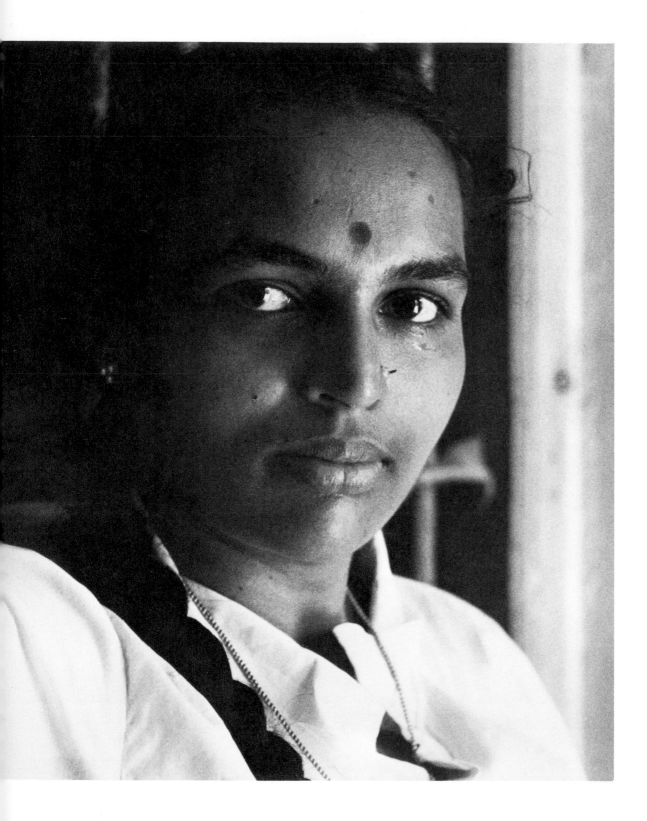

Who is Vanita?
Woman.
One
and many.

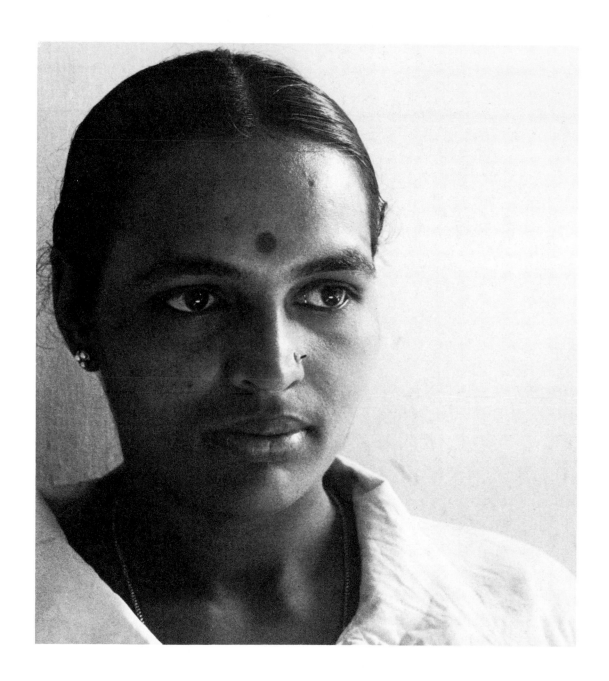

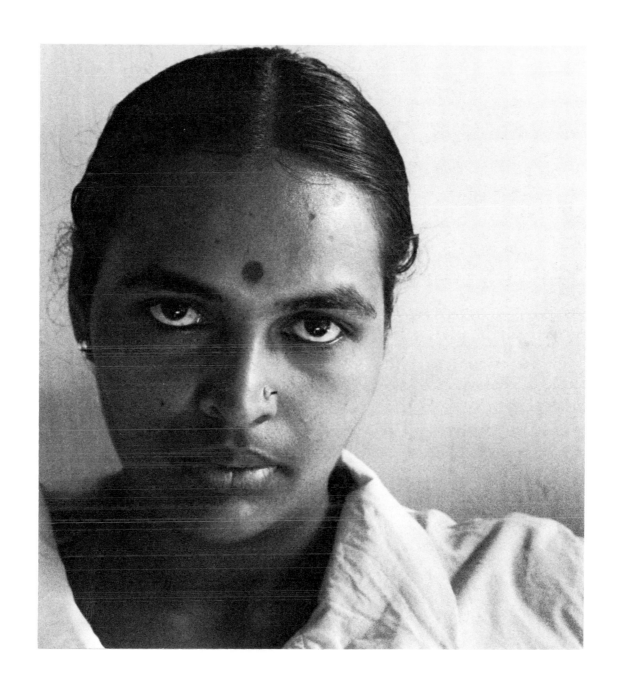

Beauty and its mystery

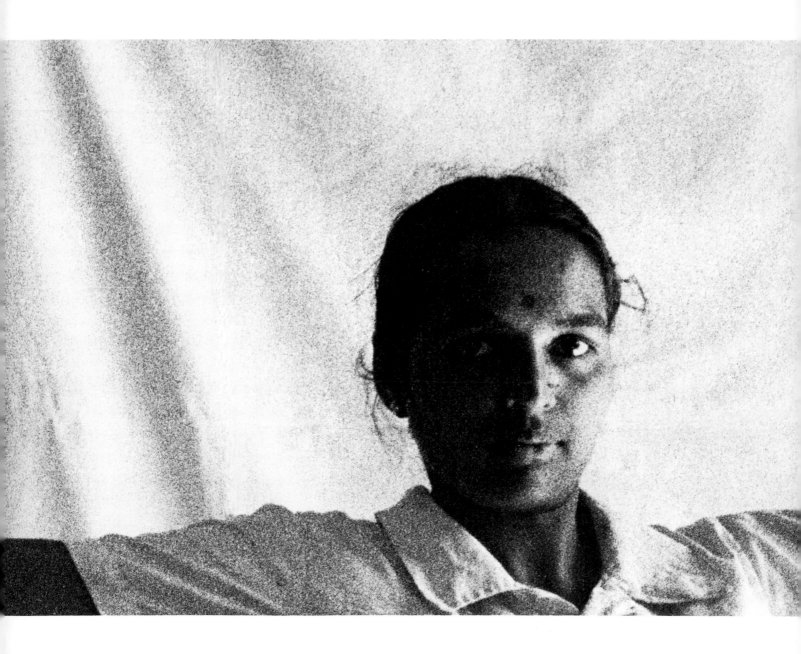

Who is Vanita?
She is Kali. She is Durga.
She is India.

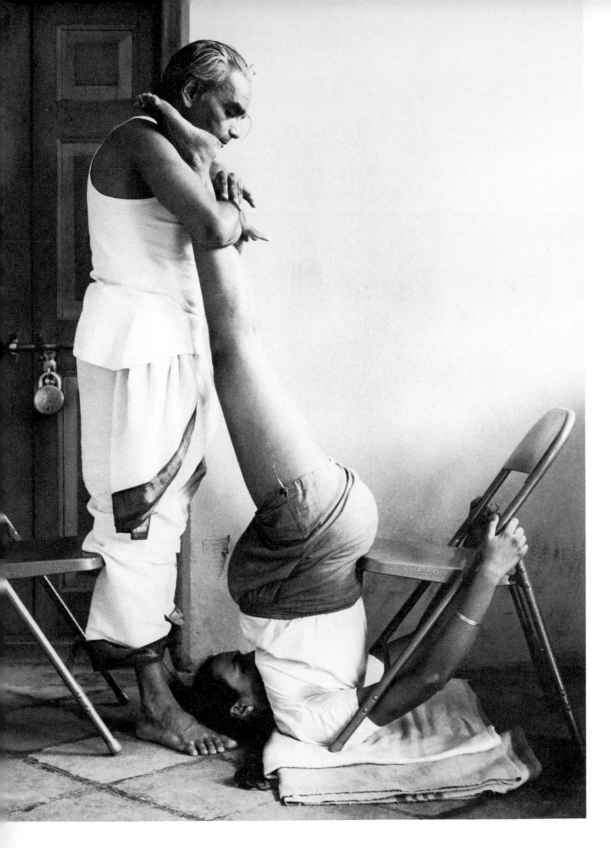

Perfect knowledge in the Guru,
complete confidence in the śiṣya.

Vanita is the second daughter of B. K. S. Iyengar, a "student of Yoga," as he modestly likes to call himself.

In fact, he is a perfect exponent of this ancient, purely traditional Indian art.

His students are as numerous as some of them are famous.

The great Yehudi Menuhin is one of them.

Many others are royal.

But whoever is devoted and sincerely wants to learn, whether old or young, rich or poor, great or humble, may come and work with him.

For years, without ever missing once, except when he is on world tours, invited by his many students abroad, this great teacher has conducted group classes in Bombay on Saturdays and Sundays.

Year in, year out, you can always see him at the Campion School, for he is, indeed, as punctual as the sun.

Like any good Master, B. K. S. Iyengar is an exacting man who will always ask of you far more than you ever thought you could do.

He will teach you that perfection is not for man

since however good you thought your own practice was, he will show you how to improve it!

And that there is, indeed, no end to improvement!

Indeed, you must be brave, not to say bold, to become the student of this terrible and yet deeply kind man who relentlessly will keep spurring you ever closer to what is right.

And will take you beyond what you always took to be your poor limitations.

But then, I can truthfully say, you will never regret it.

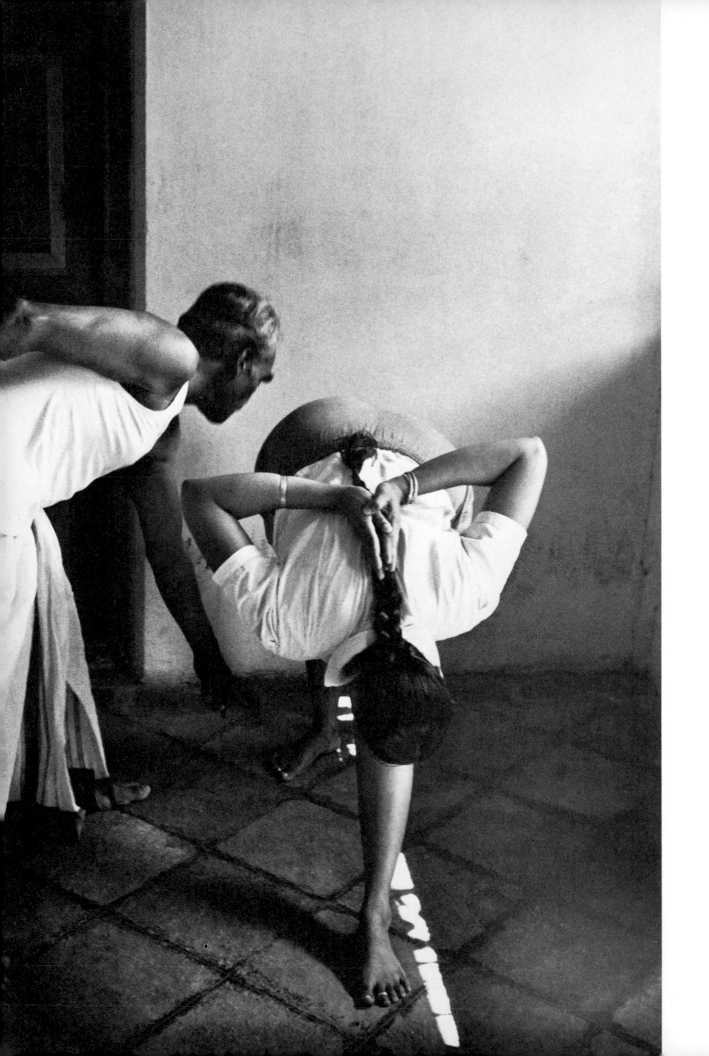

By the way,
no one in this family
ever touches
meat or fish
or eggs or cheese.
According to our scientists
with their famous
protein-need,
all these people
ought to be dead!
Or at least very, very
weak . . .

Strange . . .

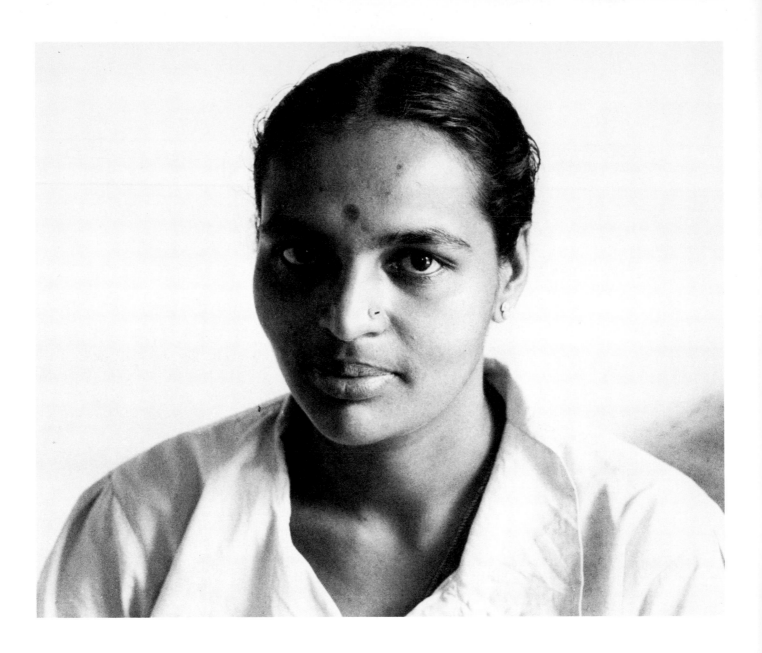

All the pictures in this book were taken, of course, in Poona.
One beautiful morning.
Slowly, quietly, peacefully,
one Asana evolving from another.
Like ripples
on the sweet face of a mountain lake
which a gentle breeze
makes suddenly shiver
and smile.
Like pearls
linked to one another
by the golden, secret thread
of breath.

Yes, it was a perfect day.
A perfect, unique moment.
And it was a rare privilege
to capture it
and make it last.

For such a joy
the author, once again,
wishes to express his deep gratitude
both to Vanita and to her father.

and a few days later

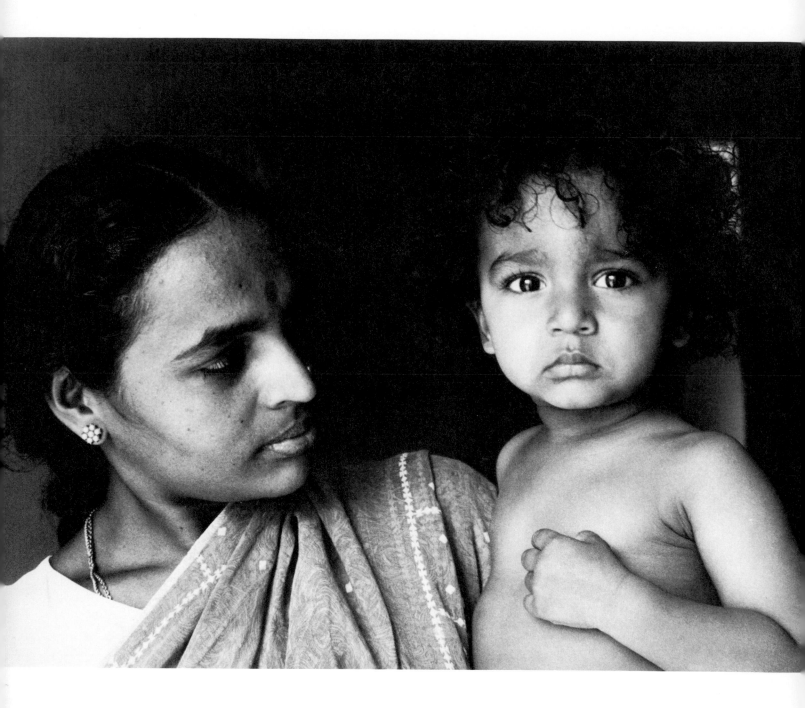

And a few days later . . .
When was that?
A year ago!
It seems it was yesterday
that Kautchik was born.
At home, of course,
in the most natural, easiest way.
Fast, indeed, fast flies
the cruel arrow of time!

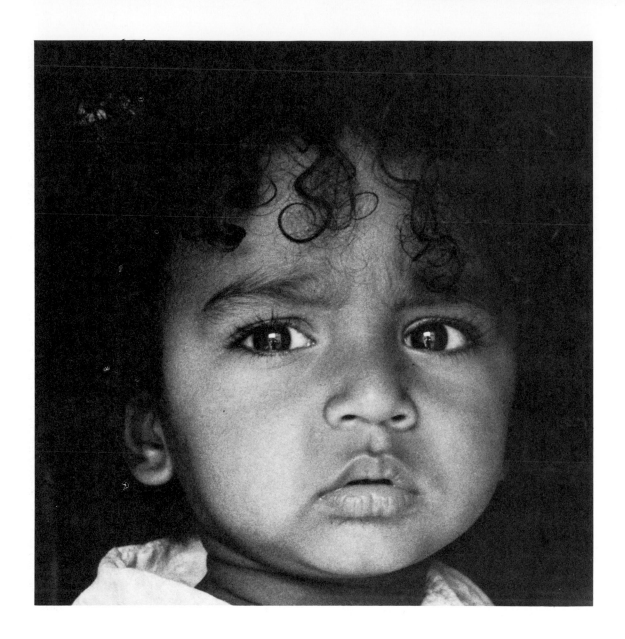

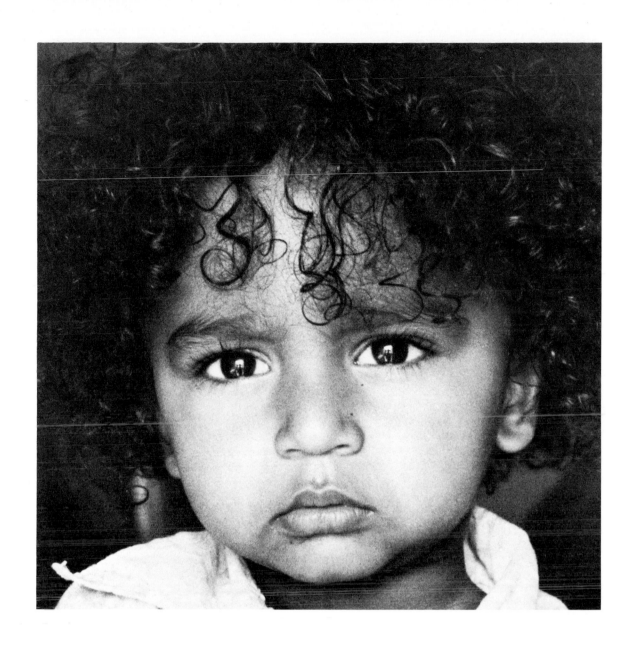

A boy!
Out of my own flesh and blood!

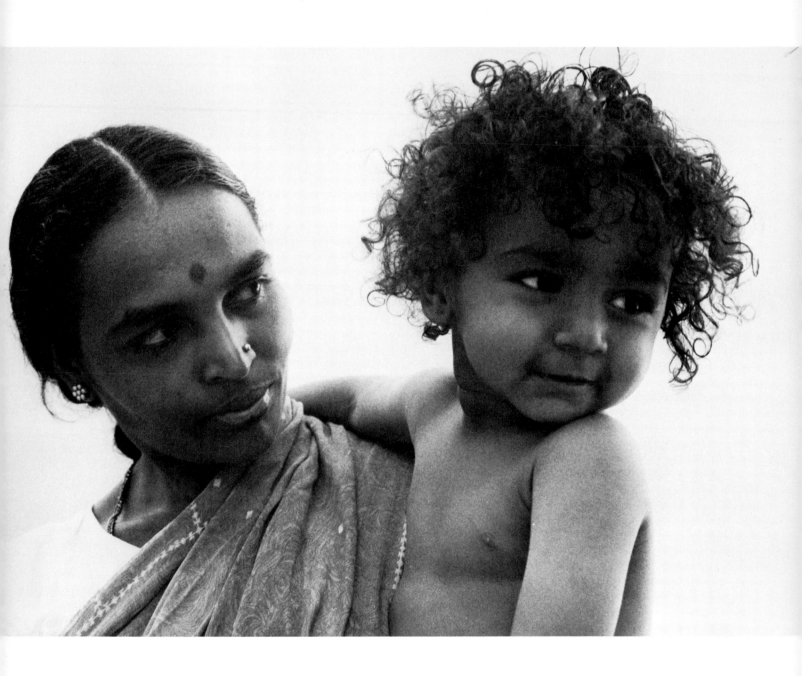

I will die?
No. *I* will grow, grow
until *I* overflow.

A maiden dies.
A child is born.
A maiden dies
and the next moment smiles
reborn as a mother.

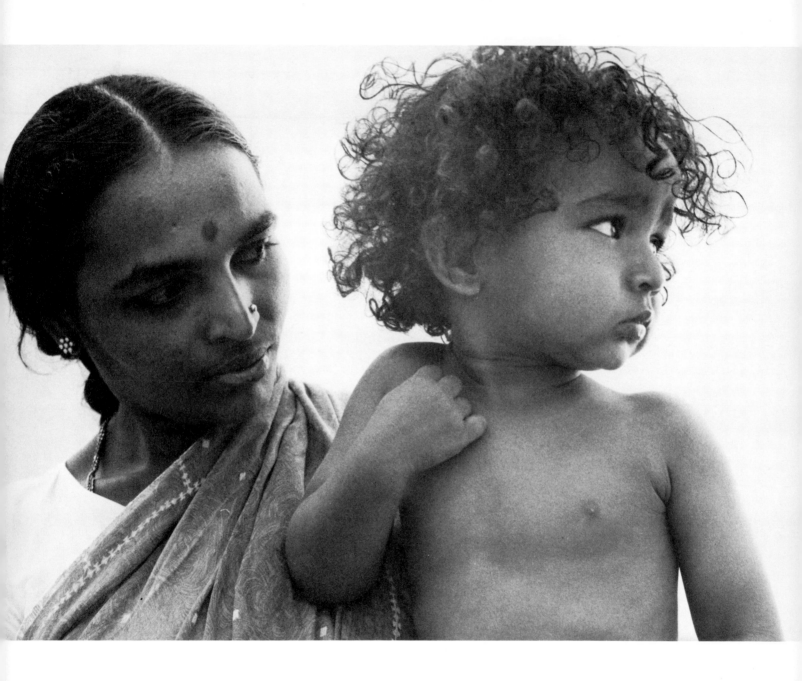

One becomes two.
Mother *and* child.
Love is born.
So is sorrow.

farewell

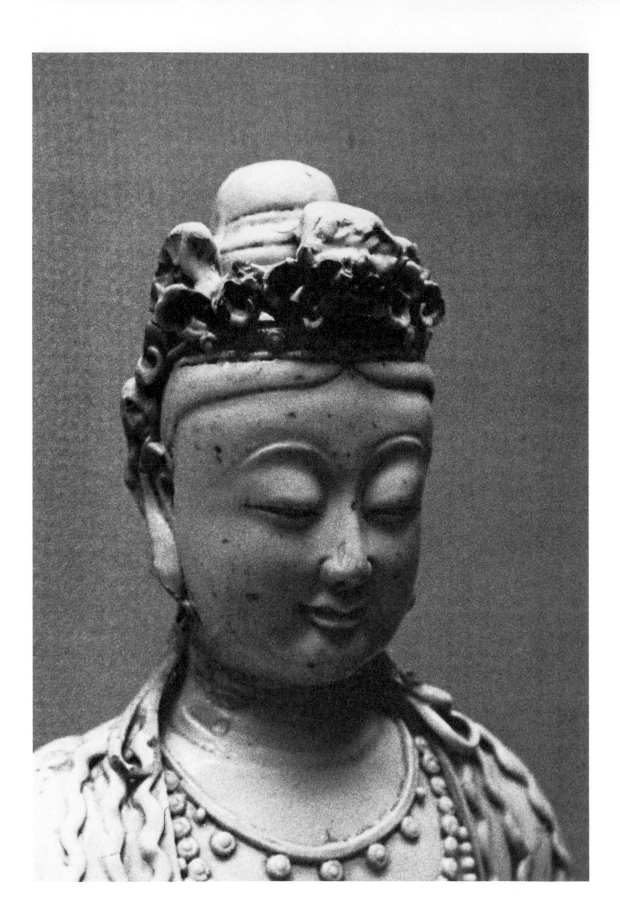

If you think:
yes, I know.
How little, indeed,
are you aware that you don't know
the true nature of Brahma.

What is Brahma in you,
what is Brahma in the gods
only your heart will tell you.

—Kena Upanishad

Is there no love
free from sorrow?
Do all lights
cast a shadow?
This perfection, this bliss,
which great artists all through the ages
have been trying to capture and render,
is it a dream,
the mere creation of their distracted minds?

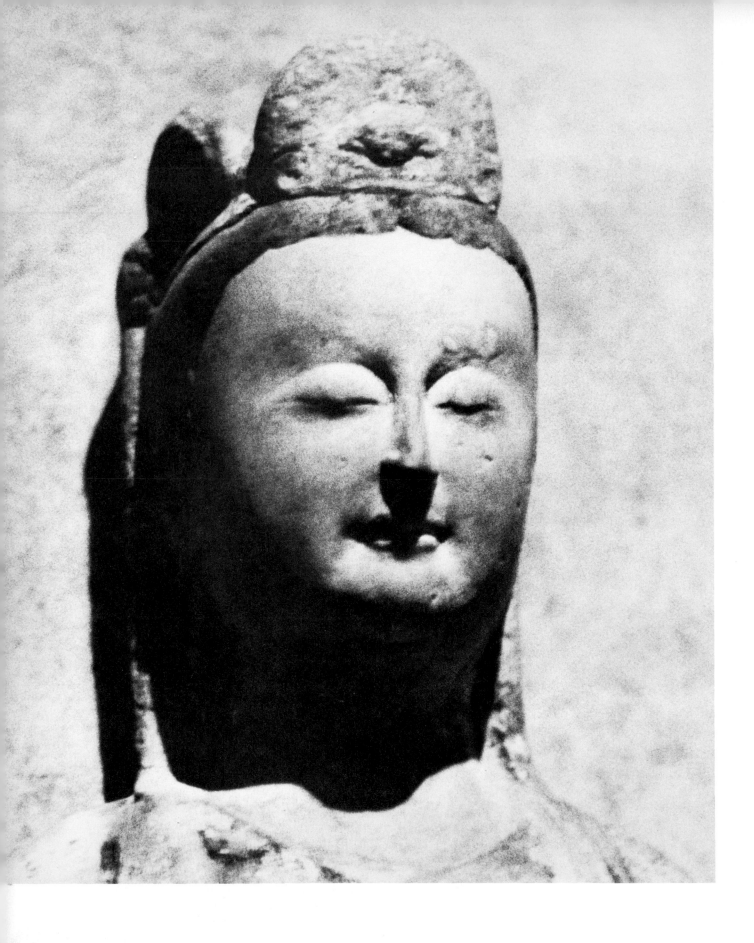

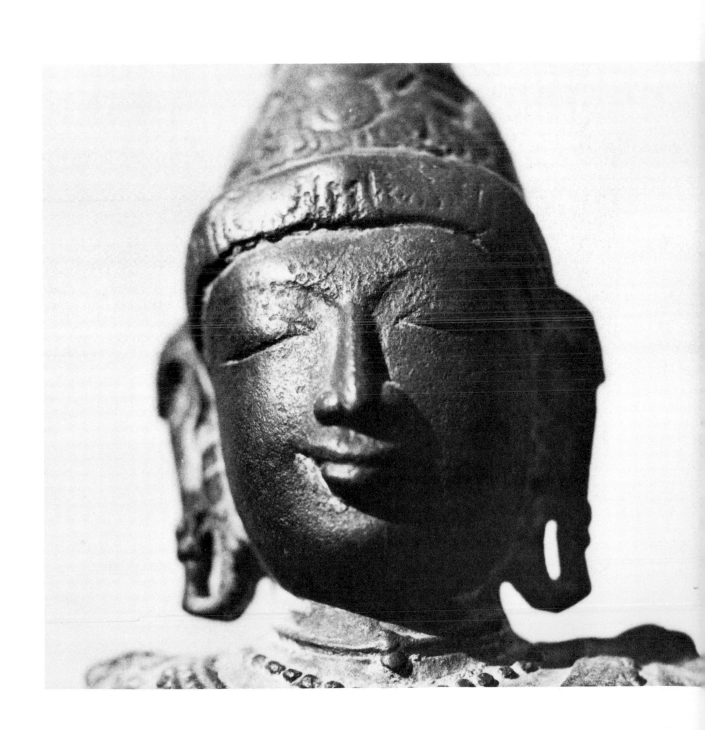

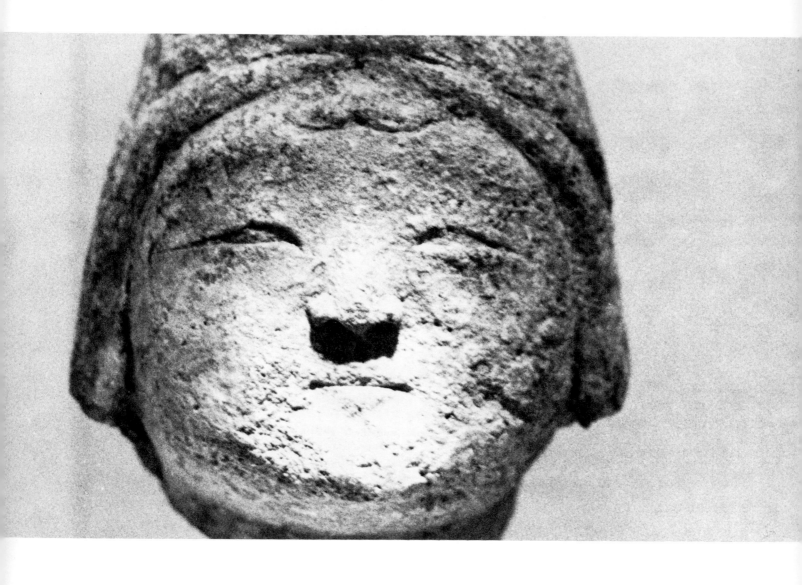

Silence!
No, it is not a dream.
Uncontaminated joy does exist:
the joy of giving
endlessly.
As do the sun,
the earth.
As does any mother.

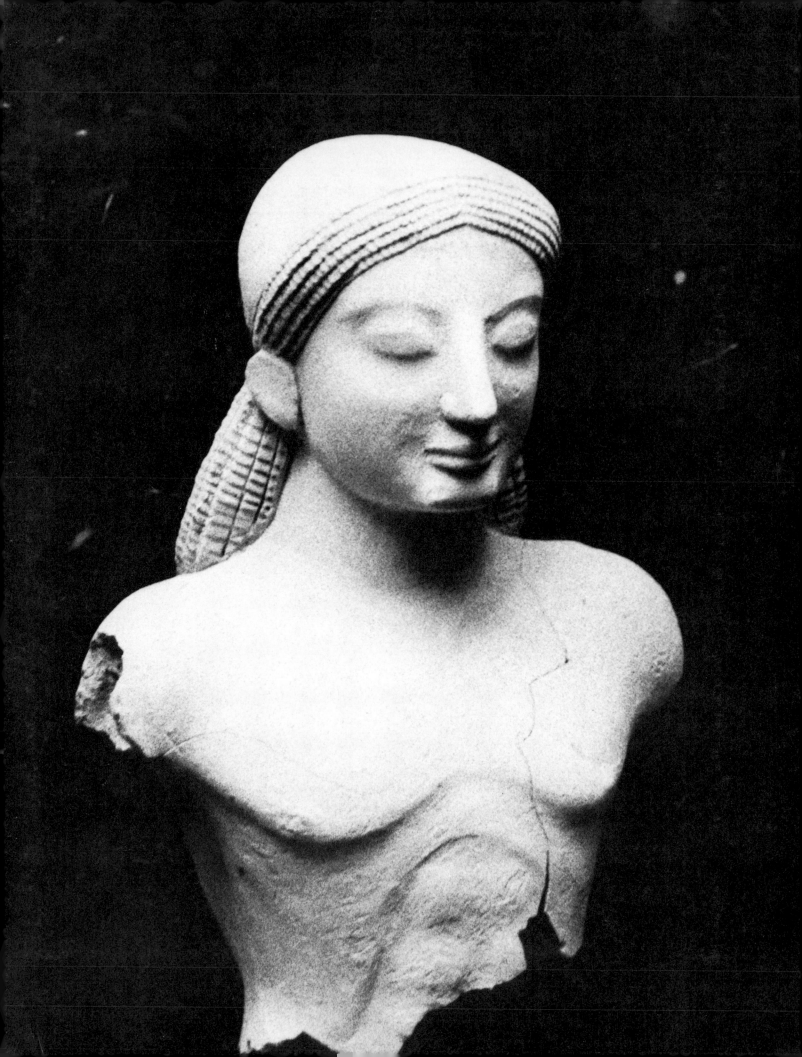

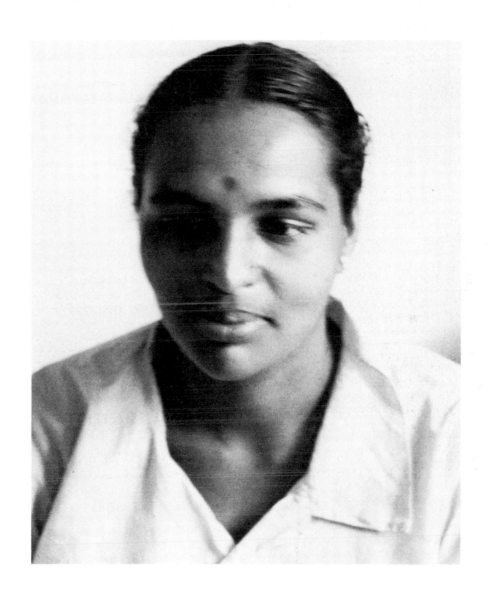

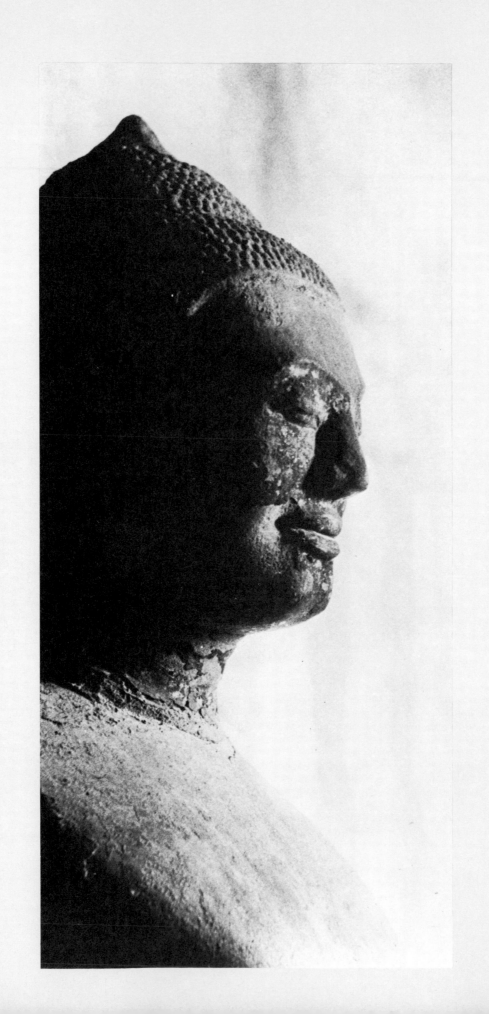

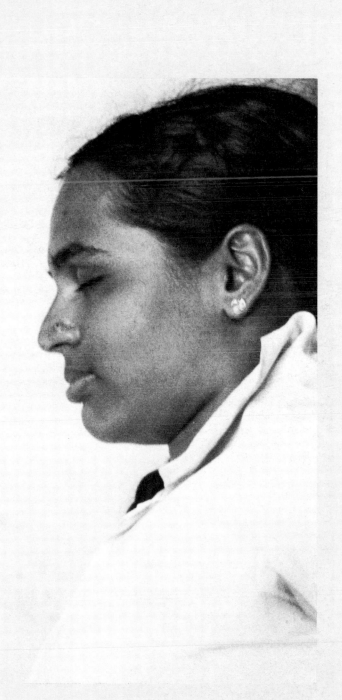

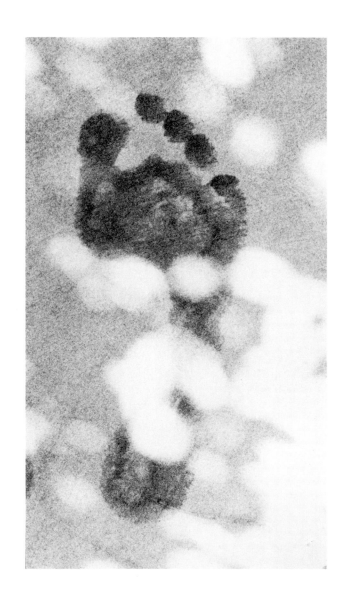

Sageness within,
Kingliness without.

A Note on the Type

The text of this book was set in film in a type face called Helvetica.
Designed by M. Miedinger in the 1950s in Switzerland and named for its
country of origin, Helvetica is perhaps the most widely accepted and
generally acclaimed sans-serif face of all time.

Composed by the Clarinda Company, Clarinda, Iowa, and
TypoGraphics Communications, Inc., New York, New York
Printed and bound by Murray Printing Company, Westford, Massachusetts